TRAVELING THERAPIST GUIDE FOR HEALTHCARE PROFESSIONALS

-Staying Sane on the Road-

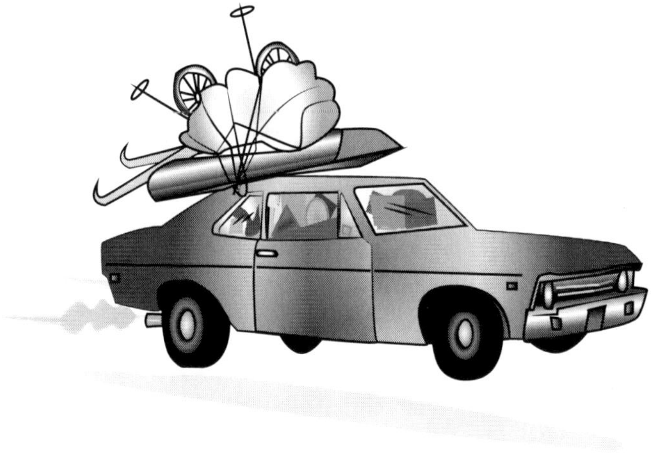

Michelle Schaefer

Cover, design, and illustrations by Michelle Schaefer, Bohemian Spirit Design.

ISBN: 9780615943244

Bohemian Spirit Design
1305 N. H Street, Suite A #198
Lompoc, CA 93436
michelle@bohemianspiritdesign.com

Bohemian Spirit Design
PUBLISHING

Acknowledgments

Thank you to my best friend and husband, Peter, without whom this book would never have been written. He is the traveling Physical Therapy Assistant and main cheerleader for this book.

A huge thank-you to my accountability writer's group, Gina Black and Wanda Toro. Thank you, guys, for keeping me on task.

Preface

This book is intended for anyone thinking of starting or restarting a career in the traveling healthcare field, as well as for those already established in this career. This entire book covers information that will be helpful for folks in all traveling therapy fields, from radiology to nursing. Special emphasis has been placed on traveling physical therapy in order to write from our direct experience and to fill a missing niche.

On that note, welcome to your new adventure! I've worked to create a book that covers all you'll need to know, while being easy to read and fun. I've included words of wisdom throughout from my husband, Peter, so you'll get firsthand information from a traveling Physical Therapy Assistant (PTA). This book encompasses five years of our traveling research, with Peter working as the PTA and me as the research, development, online student, and get-an-interesting-job-wherever-we landed other half.

This traveling program has been a wonderful experience for both my husband and me, and we wish you all the best!

—Michelle Schaefer

Contents

Part C - Preparing for Your New Assignment

I'm Official! Now What?

Your New Digs

Getting the Lay of the Land - Fun Stuff

Part D - Packing Up & Moving Out

What Should You Pack?

Expediting the Move-Out Process

Part E - Fun Stuff from the Road

Travelog

How to Use This Book

Each part of this book is full of stand-alone information, and for this reason some information will be repeated in different sections. This stand alone-aspect allows for a quick reference on specific topics. If you're new to traveling therapy or just love an 'exciting' read, then I suggest digesting this book from cover to cover—otherwise, just feel free to jump around as needed.

The first bit of information is the Time Line. This Time Line is a quick overview of what needs to be done and in what order to smoothly expedite the process. Each aspect of the Time Line will be covered in more depth on the following pages.

Time Line

This is a general time line. Feel free to adjust things as needed. In general, it's good to give yourself a month, at the very least, to plan and organize for your first assignment.

Starting Out … 1-2 Months before Assignment

- ❑ Research traveling therapy companies
- ❑ **Give notice to your current job, home, utilities,etc.**
- ❑ Research locations and traveling companies
- ❑ **Get passport photos made (for applications)**
- ❑ Fill out travel company application
- ❑ **Plan your move and alert friends and family**
- ❑ Set up mail-forwarding program (if needed)
- ❑ **Gather your housing references**
- ❑ Get vehicle checked out and vehicle insurance in order
- ❑ **Make copies of important papers. Leave them with family/friends**
- ❑ Get TB and urine tests (your recruiter will schedule this for you)
- ❑ **Check to make sure your CPR certification is current**

Get Ready … 2-4 Weeks before

- ❑ Find a location
- ❑ **Apply for license, if you don't already have one for that state**
- ❑ Get a haircut (if needed)
- ❑ **Interview (usually by phone) with new facility**

Get Set … 1-2 weeks before

- ❑ Sign contract
- ❑ **Fill out more paperwork for the facility**
- ❑ Research your new home
- ❑ **Plan how you will find housing**
- ❑ Pack (goes quickly if you've already planned what to pack)

Woohoo! You're There! … 1- 7 days before

- ❑ Head to your new home, unpack, and set up
- ❑ **Drive by the new facility and meet the staff**
- ❑ Enjoy your first day of work

Respect the Adjustment Period & Have Fun!

Part A
Research

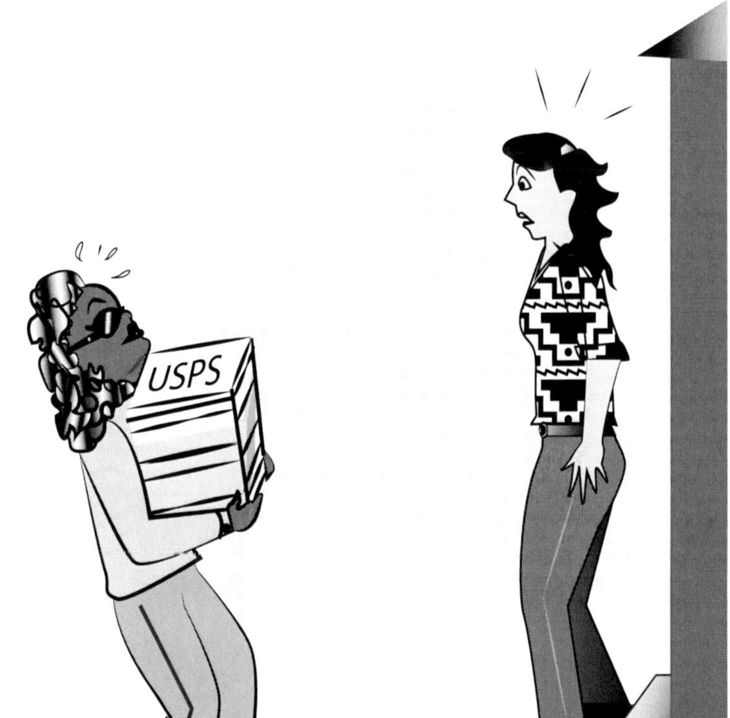

Research - Paperwork - Research

The Lowdown on Traveling Therapy

1

- What Is a Traveling Therapist?
- Why become a Traveling Therapist?
- Types of Traveling Companies

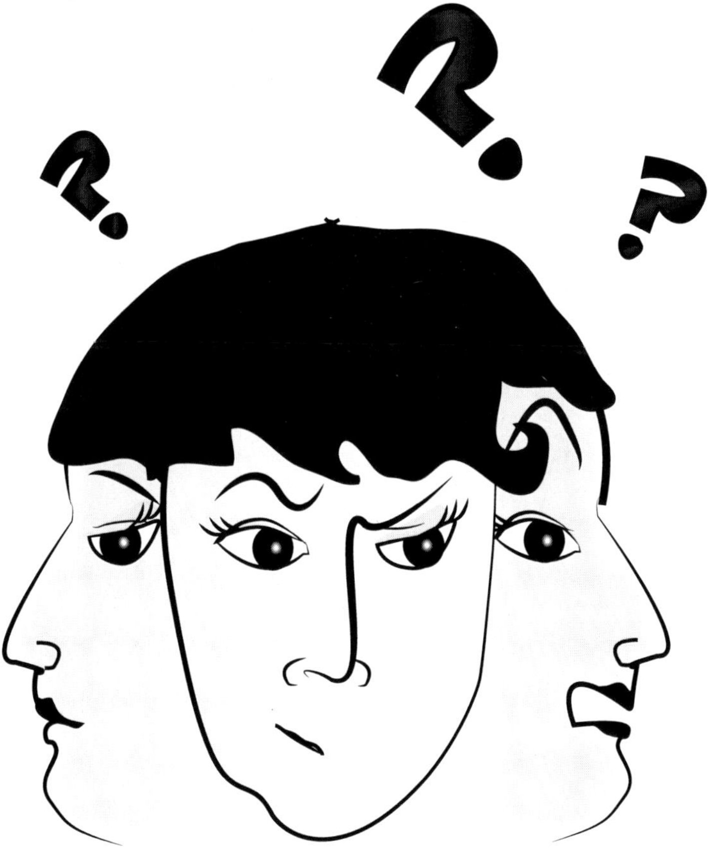

Chapter 1

▸ What Is a Traveling Therapist?

The majority of information covered herein will be helpful for all types of traveling healthcare providers, including nurses, although a traveling 'therapist' generally implies someone in the allied healthcare fields. Health care providers who are not in the nursing, medical, or pharmaceutical industries are called allied healthcare providers. The allied health profession generally covers: physical therapists, physical therapy assistants, occupational therapists, certified occupational therapist assistants, speech language pathologists, respiratory therapists, and select radiology professionals.

In researching what 'legally' constitutes the term 'traveling therapist', I had to dig deep, as many traveling companies were a bit vague about the meaning. They knew just enough to keep themselves in the clear. You, however, will need to know a bit more to stay on good terms with the IRS. Yes, the IRS has and does occasionally audit travelers. Rarely have I heard of a traveler being audited, but it's never fun to be the statistic. Out-of-compliance travelers may have to return their tax benefits and stipends for the year(s) they were not in compliance.

The IRS sees therapists as official travelers if they travel more than 50 miles from their home base and work less than one year (including vacations and breaks) in one area, with no plans to continue working there. Anyone not meeting the federal guidelines as a traveling therapist may be considered an itinerant worker and thus not be allowed the same tax benefits and stipends.

One tax company that regularly works with travelers said they'd only had a few audits over the years. Most came back fine, but two travelers were found to be out of compliance and one was required to pay back one year of tax benefits. It may not happen often, but it'll hurt in the pocketbook if it happens to you.

What constitutes my home base?

Your recruiter will give you a form to fill out, stating that you have a tax home base that is the hub from which you travel. Some travelers may list a parent's house for their home base. And while that works to keep your traveling company satisfied, it may not keep you fully in compliance with the IRS.

Questions you'll need to answer:

* What constitutes my home base?
* How long can my assignment last in the same location?
* How long do I need to wait before returning for an assignment in the same location?

From my research, the definition of 'full compliance' is a bit nebulous, and it appears to be up to the interpretation of the IRS. Here are a few things they will be looking for:

1. You must have lived and worked in your tax home base before starting the traveling program. In other words, you must have lived at this location for at least one year as a non-traveler before or between travel assignments.
2. You must continue to maintain your tax home base by paying rent or mortgage and maintenance fees.
3. You must show signs that you plan to return to this location by such things as car registration, bank accounts,

mailing service, election registration, and/or storage space at the address of your tax home base.

4. Epstein LaRue, in her book *Highway Hypodermics*, also mentions that "You must have either a family member using the residence, or you must use the residence frequently as lodging." and "There must be a realistic expectation that you will return to live at your claimed tax residence."

I've heard advice from travel companies that you need only follow a few of the things on this list. Still other travel companies —such as *TravelTax.com*, a company started by a former traveler— delve much deeper and have an entire page of questions for you to fill out to establish whether you indeed have a federally recognized tax home base.

How long can my assignment last?

Most recruiting companies will specify that you cannot work a full year in one location or else that location becomes your new tax home base. Thus, if you stay 365 days in one location, you'll negate your traveler status for that past year.

After talking to my tax accountant, I decided to dig deeper for more defined directives. What I found was again a bit fuzzy. It seems that, according to the IRS, you're okay to return to work at a previous location if you've been away from it for seven months and showed no plan to return to it. Some companies tell their recruits that a four-to-five-month break is fine, and still others say a three-month break is okay.

My accountant said one of her audited travelers—who'd worked elsewhere for three months and came back to the same location— was seen by the IRS not as a traveler but instead as an itinerant worker. The federal government counted those three months away simply as vacation time and added it to the time she had worked. She therefore had worked over her allotted time and had to repay tax breaks and stipends. Some travelers don't worry about the risks, while others follow the rules to the letter. I tend to err on the side of safety.

Tax information

All of the previous questions regarding what is 'federally legal and allowable' bring up another subject: taxes. It's often a good idea to find a tax company specializing in traveling therapists or a specific accountant at the firm who is knowledgeable in this area. The accountants we met were often more familiar with the term 'traveling nurse', but it wasn't much of a stretch for them to come up to speed with the legalities for a traveling therapist. Often the main difference was whether or not one itemized deductions.

▸ Why become a Traveling Therapist?

Benefits:

1. Great Pay –Tax-free federal benefits
2. Adventure
3. Cultural Incentives

Downsides:

1. Leaving your home, family, and friends
2. Relocating often
3. Regularly jumping into new facilities and different ways of doing things

Actually, the downside of traveling is only a downside if you're not drawn to it. Otherwise it's simply a great adventure. Not everyone is in a place in their lives where this direction calls to them, and that's why the government gives incentives to the rest of us—well, that plus the fact that we have to maintain two home locations.

▸ Types of Traveling Companies

Traveling therapy companies are staffing companies that market you and contract directly with the healthcare facilities or with the healthcare facilities' own contracted staffing company. Often they will market you to specific facilities—those with which they have a working relationship. However, they are usually open to putting in the extra time to create relationships with new facilities in locations in which you are interested. The terms 'travel company', 'recruiter', and 'recruiting agency' all refer to the travel companies and their staff.

Smaller Staffing Company

A 'smaller staffing company' might be smaller in size or simply smaller in their geographical scope. Instead of working on a national level, they may only contract within a few counties, a single state, or a grouping of states. The benefits of a smaller-sized staffing company are that they can sometimes, though not always, give you more one-on-one time and support. They'll also often have strong relationships with facilities in their chosen area. This may make it easier for you to win that contract. So if you're only interested in working within a small area of the country, give a good look at these staffing companies.

National Staffing Company

National staffing companies have contracts and relationships with facilities all over the country. The larger companies often have specific recruiters for different areas of the country. Some companies will allow you to stay with your original recruiter no matter where you travel. This can be helpful if you've created a good connection with your recruiter. Others may hand you over to a different recruiter who has a better working knowledge of the area where you'd like to work.

Regardless of what kind of travel company you decide to use, make sure they meet your criteria and that they have good follow-through. The size doesn't matter as much as the support and the bottom line—and neither small nor large travel companies corner the market on these. You'll want to do your homework.

Finding your Traveling Therapy Company

2

- How to Find a Travel Company
- What to Look and Ask For
- What to Watch Out For
- What to ask Yourself before Changing Your Current Company

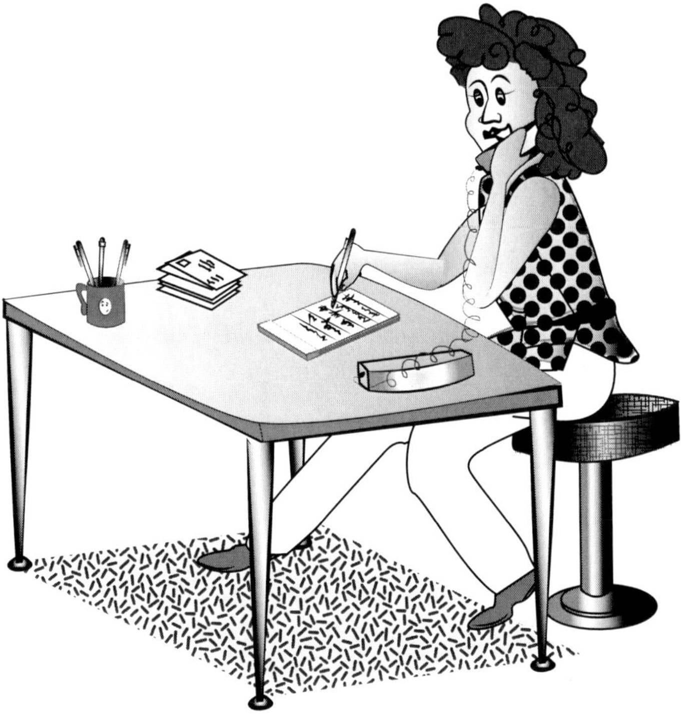

▸ How to Find a Travel Company

Call around

Hit the phones to talk with and interview different agencies. Ask the questions we've listed throughout this chapter and compare each company's answer. It's important to remember that the recruiter's job is to recruit you, while your job is to sift through the emotional tug to get to the basics. Some recruiters will make things sound better than they actually are to get you to sign on with them.

To find different travel companies or have them find you, post your resume on consolidated staffing company websites (if you want a lot of calls) and/or email/call companies you find online, in magazines, or through word of mouth.

Research online and with coworkers

Check the Better Business Bureau's website to find each company's ratings and history, and talk to other travelers. Get different opinions on the same company, for sometimes a problem may have been with a particular recruiter and not with the company.

Sign up with a few different companies, or at least start relationships with up to five to get a feel for what each of them offer and how approachable they are. Sometimes one company will be great, but then your recruiter leaves and their replacement isn't so great. It can also work the other way around, so it's not always the company that's the issue. Sometimes the gifts or challenges stem from the recruiter.

Starting out as a traveler can be very intimidating, especially if you're leaving a comfortable home and a well-paying job with benefits. A good recruiter will help it all go smoothly, from paperwork to general support.

One recruiter we really liked (he eventually moved on) stayed in contact with us regularly even after we'd signed the contracts. Between assignments, he'd listen to us and try to find an assignment to our specifications, and he would email us fun facts and information on the areas we'd be driving through. Along with information on our new locations, he'd add fun tidbits related by other traveling therapists.

You won't even realize how much a recruiter is doing for you if they're good. You'll simply notice that all is going smoothly, and you won't feel as though you're floundering.

▸ What to Look and Ask For

Before calling around, first make a list of information you want to find out from the prospective company. Here is a good starting place:

1. Do they have openings or contracts/relationships in the places where you want to work?
2. Do they seem helpful and supportive?
3. Do they get back to you right away?
   Our first recruiter captured our attention and retained us because she called us back immediately and pretty much held our hand through the process. She knew that starting this new way of life was pretty strange and overwhelming, so she was there every step of the way.
4. How do their pay scales, benefit packages, and reimbursements measure up?
5. Do they offer a rewards program?

6. Do they offer health insurance? What type, and how much will it cost?
7. Do they offer a matching 401k, and how long before they start matching?
8. Do they have paid holidays and/or Personal Time Off (PTO) and/or sick days?
9. Do they pay travel expenses?
10. Do they offer bonuses (which get taxed very high)?
11. Do they allow you to find your own housing and reimburse you for this?
12. What kind of annual training do they require (beyond state-required CEUs)?

▸ What to Watch For

Pushy or intimidating recruiters

Trust how you feel, not just what you hear them saying.

Our first company was great until our recruiter left. Over the following year, we had three different recruiters. They started aggressively pushing locations and assignments on us that they knew we weren't interested in. Even as we began feeling harried, intimidated, and overwhelmed we stuck with the company we were familiar with. When we finally decided to call around and interview other companies, we found that this way of recruiting was not the status quo. Instead, we found companies/recruiters who were very helpful and sensitive to us.

Notice if the recruiter is trying to push you into an area or job that you're not interested in. Is the recruiter sensitive to your being overwhelmed at starting this new venture?

Bait and Switch

Are they telling you one thing yet putting something else in your contract?

Always, always read your contract completely

BEFORE you sign it!

▸ What to Ask Yourself before Changing Your Current Company

It's good to chat with other travelers about their travel companies but don't always take what they say at face value. Do your research. When we found out that another traveler seemed to be getting more from their travel company even though they had less experience, we decided to look into expanding our horizons.

Don't allow yourself to be fooled when you're looking for contract openings online. Many companies list the places they have relationships with, not necessarily ones that currently have openings.

When talking with other companies, some sounded so wonderful and sincere, yet we were left still wondering if they'd sold us a line—sometimes they had.

Don't get drawn to leave your present traveling company by a sweet-talking recruiter doing a snow job on you.

Instead of changing companies immediately, we took the information we gleaned from our research to our present traveling company. They ended up working with us and made us an offer that worked. There was, of course, some annoyance on our part as to why these options had not been offered previously. In truth, the recruiters are doing their job for the same reason as the traveler—to make money.

The moral of this story is, if you like your present recruiter/company, then try working out the financial stuff with them. It's easier than filling out the mountains of paperwork for another company. Plus, you may lose your matching 401k only to find out that the new company has even more hoops to jump through.

Unless you ask for it, you probably won't get it handed to you even from a helpful recruiter.

A few reasons you might want to change your traveling company:

1. **Financial mismanagement**
   Always always check your pay stubs against hours worked. Compare your hours worked and pay promised. We once had to go back and research a whole year to get payment that we'd been shorted.
2. **Better incentives**
3. **No contracts in the area you want to work**
   Even if you find out that your company doesn't have a working relationship with a certain facility, see if they can create one before you give up on them. This some times takes a month or so even if the facility is open to it. Some Skilled Nursing Facilities (SNFs) and hospitals work with many recruiting companies, and some only with a few.

Where Do You Want to Work?

3

- Type of Facility
- Size of Town and Facility
- Geographical Location
- Other Preferences to Factor

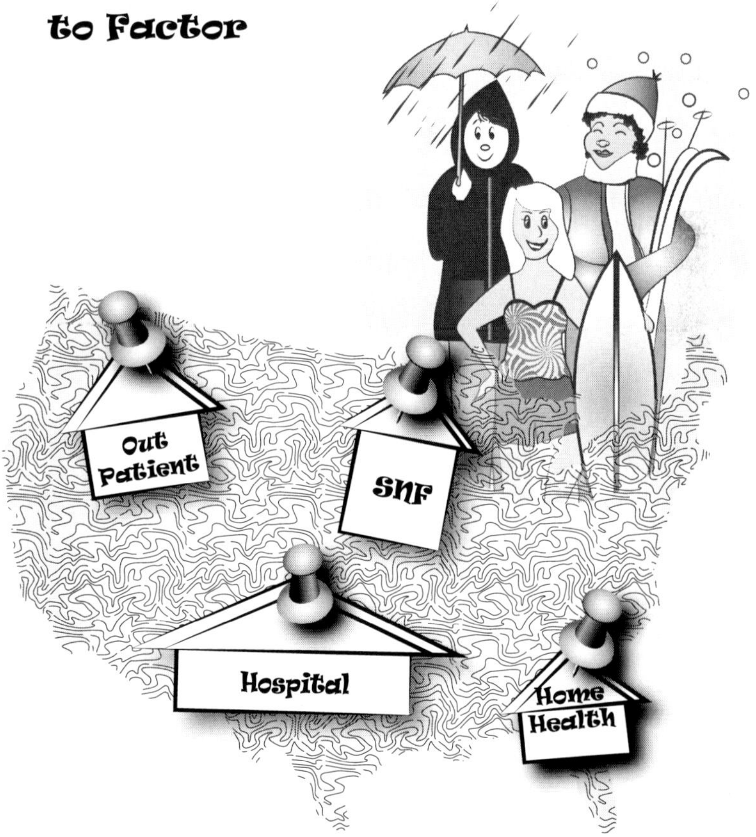

▸ Facility Type

Each facility type has its own strengths and challenges. You may want to stick with the one you're familiar with or take on something new.

Along with different types of facilities, it's important to look at the quality of the facilities. Many are great; some aren't run very well; and still others may simply be financially strapped. These aren't huge issues if you're signing on for only a thirteen-week assignment, but they may be important factors if you've signed on for a longer contract. Thus, if you have concerns about the quality of your prospective location, it's a good idea to first sign on for the minimum contract and then extend it as desired. One traveler said he had to make equipment for the patients at one facility by borrowing pieces off old neglected parts, and at another facility he witnessed patient neglect. These issues are rare, but they're something to keep in mind.

Whenever you change facility types, it's a good idea to brush up on the new one. When in **outpatient**, you might want to carry a few reference books with you, as the patients might want to know the exact whys and what-fors and names for each thing you do; whereas at the **nursing homes,** you might need to step back and go more with the flow of the patients.

Mix it up! Changing to different types and sizes of facilities will keep things fresh. Plus, it'll be a marketable addition to your résumé.

Inpatient hospitals are often more regimented than outpatient facilities but the therapies are more routine. If you like to see a higher level of progress and a quicker turnover of patients, then hospitals may be right up your alley. Some facilities may also give you the option of doing home health.

Outpatient is a bit more challenging, knowledge-wise, as you're often confronted with something new every day, yet the atmosphere may be less regimented than inpatient hospitals.

Skilled Nursing Facilities (SNFs) are rewarding if you're interested in a (usually) more relaxed atmosphere, with more time to get to know your patients/residents, although at some SNFs the productivity expectations may be higher. You'll also experience a bit of an adjustment changing from higher level functioning patients at the hospital and outpatient facilities to lower level functioning patients at SNFs. However, the rewards of really making a connection with residents in the relaxed atmosphere can be a wonderful change.

Home Health is another interesting option that some facilities offer. Make sure you have a good idea of the community and awareness of your surroundings, as you'll be going into unfamiliar areas and homes. We have a friend who does this work exclusively and really enjoys it, but she had to get lost more than a few times to get her bearings. Some therapists don't feel drawn to home health, especially many females working alone, although some companies make sure to send two therapists at a time.

Make sure your contract states the mile radius of your assignment. One traveler had to travel a radius of 60-plus miles in the San Francisco Bay Area for home health. Whether this is your favorite or least favorite travel job option, make sure your contract stipulates how you'll be paid (by the hour or visit) and if they pay mileage and travel time.

▸ Size of Town and Facility

A larger facility will often be faster paced than a smaller one and is sometimes more cutting edge, although occasionally opposite can be true. For example, there was a more relaxed atmosphere at a large hospital in Santa Fe, New Mexico, than there was at a small outpatient clinic in Santa Barbara, California.

It's good to interview therapists from the facility you're going to, since no rules are hard and fast, and you'll want to know what you're getting into.

▸ Geographical Location

When deciding on which geographical area to work in there are multiple things to think about. Some people focus on just going where the money is, as many people travel to pay off debt. Whether that leads them out in the boonies or to the big city, they don't mind. Others want to travel near friends, the ski slopes, tourist areas, etc. And still others blend the two by setting aside one assignment a year to work in a higher-paying area, no matter where it takes them.

We've done a mix of these, but mostly we like to go to smaller, rustic touristy towns—especially in their off-seasons. They usually have the energy and vibrancy from the tourist cash flow, without the weekday traffic. We do a lot of research before we give our recruiter specific areas where we'd like to go, and they call around for us.

It can be helpful to take your first assignment close to your home base. This way you can go back and visit or pick up things you might have forgotten.

Travelers are often in high demand during the holidays, as many take time off to be with family, leaving vacancies in the field. Thus, if you want to work during this time yet still celebrate with loved ones, check for an opening near your family for the holiday season. Otherwise, you can simply take your pick from the multiple openings and even take advantage of holiday sign-on bonuses. However, remember that bonuses do get taxed at a much higher rate so work out the math rather than simply getting taken in by the idea of a big bonus.

Helping your recruiter help you

Give your recruiter the parameters you want, then look up their proposed sites on places like visitor bureau sites, chambers of commerce, *hometownlocator.com*, *city-data.com*, etc.

▸ Finding Location Information

You can go to a website like *findyourspot.com* and spend a few minutes typing in all your preferences. It'll then spit out a list of places compatible with you. It isn't always perfect, so you'll want to do more research from there, but it's a good jumping-off point.

We like *city-data.com* because it gives a good overview, including statistics and occasional forums. The chamber of commerce and visitor bureaus also have a wealth of information.

When checking statistics such as crime rates, note the difference between crimes against people as opposed to objects. Eugene, Oregon, a happening city, has few crimes against people but more than its fair share of thefts, mostly of students' bikes. For a more roundabout information search, go to *meetup.com* and see what kind of meetups are happening in the area.

See more information in Chapter 8 – Getting the Lay of the Land.

▸ Other Preferences to Factor in

There are a lot of things to factor in when looking into a location, such as outdoor activities; tourist attractions; being near friends and family; arts and culture; progressive (think college towns) or conservative areas; terrain: mountain, valley, coastal; weather: hot, cold, humid, foggy, snowy; etc.

Seasons

If you really like an area but don't like the weather, then pick a season when the weather is more to your liking.

We loved the monsoons of the Texas summers but not the annual heat and humidity. In Santa Fe, we enjoyed the earlier monsoons as well as the light snow of winter. One plan we still have is to work in beautiful New England in the fall.

Weather

Do your homework, as every state and city may have different microclimates. Even a single state like California can have many different climate zones. If you enjoy your facility, you may want to extend your stay, so it's good to check the annual weather patterns before committing to a longer contract.

Part B
Getting Started

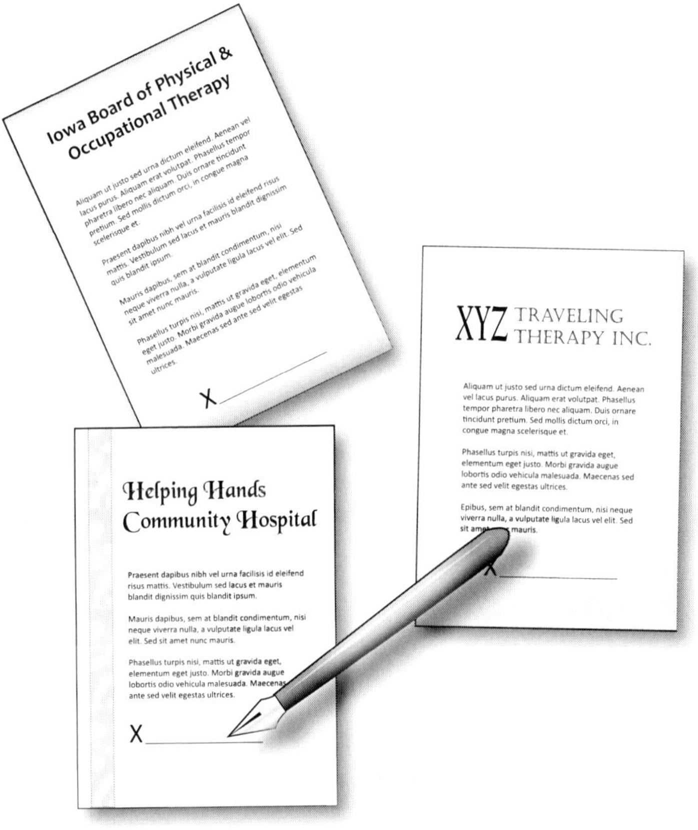

Yet more paperwork!

Becoming a Traveling Therapist 4

- **How Do I Get Started?**
- **Paperwork Needed**
  - State Licensing
  - Traveling Company
  - New Job and Job Site
- **The Site Interview**

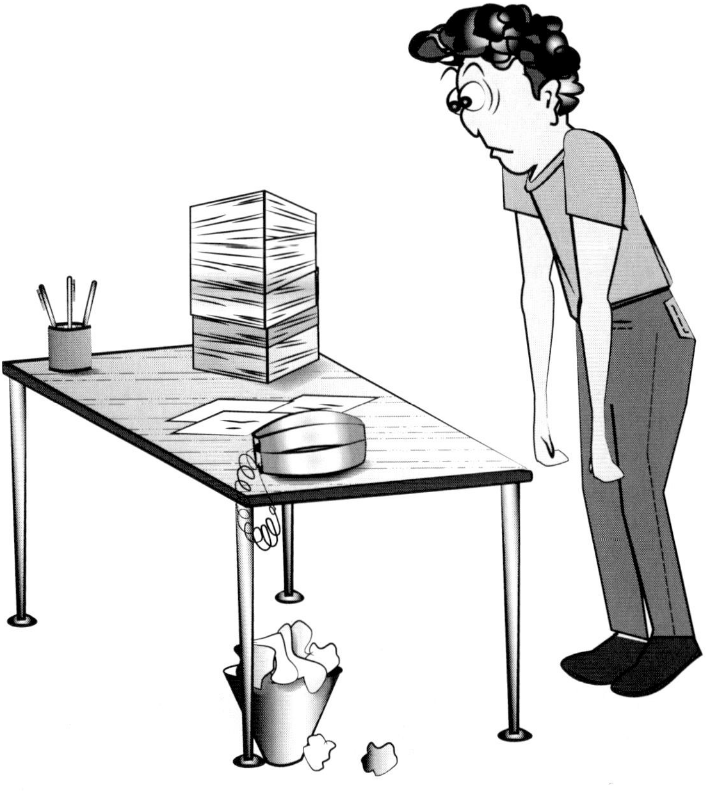

▸ How Do I Get Started?

Generally, you'll need two passport-type photos. One will be for your travel company and the other for the facility in which you'll be working. Another photo may be needed each time you sign on with a new facility; therefore, it's a good idea to have extras made. You can get your photos taken anywhere that creates passport photos.

▸ Paperwork Needed

State Licensing

The first thing you'll want to do is check to see how long it'll take to get licensed in the state(s) you want to work. Ask the recruiter to check on this. Don't expect them to already know.

Once, while working with our favorite recruiter, we left northern Washington and chased down a job in Idaho. Zipping east through Washington, past miles of grain fields, we headed for our destination, Cour d'Alene, Idaho. Three-quarters of the way there, we suddenly got a call from our recruiter—he hadn't realized it would take three months to get licensed in Idaho, as the licensing board only met quarterly (at that time). Yikes! We took it in stride, after the initial panic, as the drive was beautiful, and just used it as a re-connoiter trip for future job possibilities.

Often the recruiting agency will pay for your initial state licensing fee and annual updates but only for the state where you're currently signing a contract. If you have a lot of different state licenses, you may find yourself with a large annual outlay to keep them all up-to-date else face penalty charges when you want to reinstate them. It's all worth it if you plan to work in those states again, but it's just something to think about. If, for instance, you get licensed in Washington, Idaho, and Oklahoma but the job actually ends up being in Washington, then you'll most likely have to eat the cost of the Idaho and Oklahoma licenses.

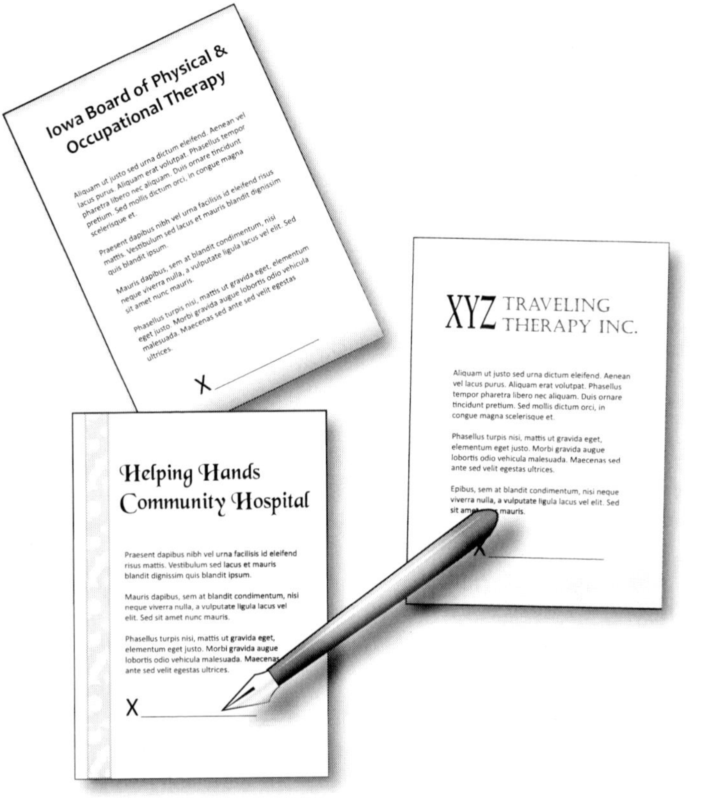

It can be helpful to have the flexibility of holding multiple licenses in which states you'll want to work as you won't have to worry about waiting to for them. Some states allow you to get your license quickly if you already hold one in a nearby state.

To find out where to get your licensing paperwork, just contact your recruiter. You can also search online with the name of your profession followed by the state in which you are applying and the word 'license.'

Traveling Company

Your traveling company will send you a new-hire packet full of information, as well as forms you'll need to fill out, including a skills checklist. They'll want to find out your experience levels in order to better market you to the facilities.

Along with the finished forms, they'll usually want a copy of your social security card, an identification photo (passport photo), copies of your current professional license and CPR credentials, letters of reference, résumé, and a copy of your driver's license. The company will call to schedule your TB and urine tests. They may ask for other things, as well, but this list is pretty standard.

New Job and Job Site

You may have to send in another photo and possibly fill out some simple paperwork for the job site where you'll be temporarily working. You'll know more about that after talking with your recruiter and after your site interview.

▸ The Site Interview

After you and your recruiter settle on a job that interests you, he or she will send your information to the facility. If they're interested, they'll ask for an interview, which is usually done on the phone. This is an opportunity for them to learn a bit about you and for you to learn about them.

In this interview, the facility manager wants to find out if you're intelligent, knowledgeable, and work well with others. Since the manager already has a full schedule, they want to hear from you that you can be on the floor, working confidently, with only a short orientation. If you've diversified your skills by working with different types of patients and facilities, this is also where your résumé will shine.

Since this is also your opportunity to find out about the facility, you'll want to have a list of questions put together before your interview.

Here's a list of example questions:

1. How big is their facility (how many beds)?
2. How many therapists are on staff? Are any of them traveling therapists?
3. What are the typical case load and productivity standards?
4. How many Medicare A and Medicare B patients will you usually have on your case load? (This medical billing status will give you an idea of you how high or low functioning your patients/residents will be.)
5. What documentation and billing programs do they use?
6. What is the typical end and start time?
7. In how many different facilities will you be working?
8. What is the dress code?

Your Contract

5

- Negotiating Your Contract
- Length of Contract
- Hours Worked
- Time Off between Contracts
- Checklist

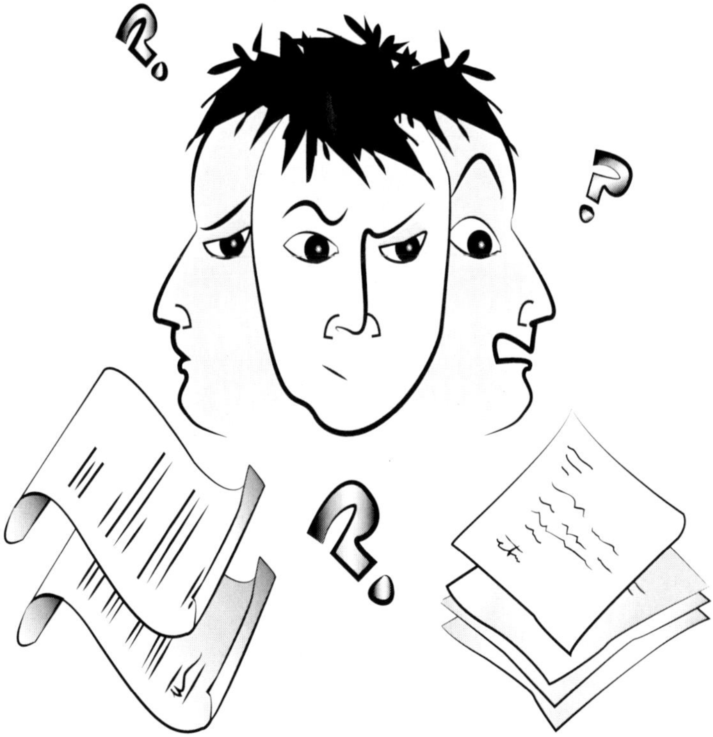

Chapter 5

▸ Negotiating Your Contract

You know you'll want good pay and quality incentives. This chapter gives you tips we've uncovered over the years for negotiating your pay as well as your tax-free stipends. You'll also need to negotiate where you'll be working, your time off, and bonuses.

Traveling Therapist's GOLDEN RULE:

Get EVERYTHING in Writing!

Your job location

It seems obvious that, if you sign a contract to work in one location, you'll be working there and not somewhere else, right? Well, that *seems* obvious, but it isn't necessarily accurate. Some companies own multiple facilities and they may want to you divide your time among them, when needed.

This can be a fun change of pace, but it can also mean a longer commute if it's in another city. Just be aware of it and make sure that it's what you want and that drive time and fuel are included in your contract.

With a contract in Eugene, Oregon, Peter was asked to work at two facilities in town as well as occasionally an hour away in another city. A different contract had him working a few weeks at a time in different locations along the Oregon coast while we stayed in a classy retirement home or at different hotels. With that contract we moved around a lot, but there was little commuting, as the facility was usually close to the hotel.

One Traveling Physical Therapist said he was verbally told he'd be working at only two facility locations. He was told he'd go to one on Monday, Wednesday, and Friday, and the second on Tuesday and Thursday. Instead, after starting the new assignment, he found himself being sent to five different facilities. Just about every day, he'd have to travel to two and sometimes three different locations.

GET IT IN WRITING!

If you prefer working in a certain facility, make sure the name of that company and the specific facility is stipulated in the contract. Just putting down the contracted company is not enough because the company may own multiple facilities.

Negotiating your pay and stipends

The basic idea is that the travel company pockets the difference between what the facility pays and what you get. Generally, the longer you're with the company and the more marketable and experienced you are, the better pay/stipends you get. A recruiter's job is to make money for their company while also supporting your needs. To that end, if you want more, you'll need to ask for it rather than wait for it to be offered.

Always be sure to get maximum tax-free per diems before negotiating your hourly pay. Your hourly pay is taxable, thus having your tax-free per diems and stipends at the federally mandated maximum and your pay at the minimum will garner you a better take-home pay.

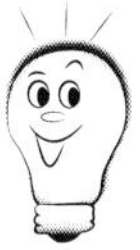

Tax-free per diems are based on Federal GSA rates. To find the maximum allowed per diems, go to *www.gsa.gov* website and type in 'per diem'. You'll then be able to choose your state and county.

Chapter 5

Know what's available.
Know what you can negotiate.

* Negotiate your hourly pay
* Negotiate your stipends (housing, clothing, vehicle, food, travel between assignments, relocation stipends, etc.)
* Negotiate your bonuses (completion, sign-on, referral)

Negotiate using your strengths.

Recruiters want to find out how easy it'll be to market you.

* Years in the profession
* Length of time you plan on being in the traveling therapy field (Companies prefer a long-term investment.)
* A solid work ethic
* Cross-training in different types of facilities
* Strong references
* Your ease of stepping into a new job
* Your ability to work well with others
* Your professionalism

Figure out what their offer boils down to.

Your recruiter will make you an offer of an hourly pay and stipends. In order to find out what your actual take-home pay boils down to, you'll need to crunch some numbers. The easiest way to do this is to make a list and divide it into two columns.

1. **Column one** – Figure out your daily take-home pay

HOURLY PAY x 8 HRS.

- TAX %	*(figure out your tax bracket)*
A	*(daily take-home wage)*

2. **Column two** – Figure out the total of your daily tax-free stipends: Write down all your monthly stipends and add them together. If your company is finding you housing* (instead of you finding your own housing), estimate the costs of rent and utilities. Don't forget to add in any bonuses you received (after subtracting the tax).

TOTAL MONTHLY STIPENDS

÷ 30 DAYS	
B	*(daily tax-free stipends)*

Calculate your actual hourly pay.

ADD A + B *(daily take home pay)*
÷ 8 HRS.

HOURLY TAKE-HOME PAY

** Note you will not actually take the housing stipend home if the facility finds your housing for you. But if you find your own housing, you will take home your housing stipend.*

Often a traveling company will take fifty cents an hour out of your pay to cover continuing education units (CEUs) without mentioning it. If you'd rather pay for your education on your own, when needed, then let them know. Otherwise you can look at it as a savings account for your CEUs and not worry about it. (That's what many travelers do.)

Chapter 5

Housing

If you find your own housing (we always have), then you'll want your hourly wage at the minimum and your per diem and allowances at the federal guideline's maximum since these are tax free.

You'll have a choice between finding your own housing or having your company find corporate housing for you. It's often less stressful to just move into an already set-up home and have all your utilities on and ready. Some folks always choose this option so they can hit the ground running when they arrive.

There are three main reasons some therapists elect to find their own housing: you'll get to control your living arrangements; you may want to be closer to your facility; and/or the place may not be well vetted by the company. The last is more of an issue in smaller communities where it's hard for the company to find suitable corporate housing.

To find out how much to negotiate for housing, if you're finding your own, check out the going rate for corporate housing in the community in which you'll be working.

Time off

In order to guarantee yourself specific days or periods of time off, you'll want to get it written in your contract.

Holiday pay

Find out your company's holiday pay and what days the facility is closed. If the facility is officially closed on a holiday—which is more likely to happen for an outpatient facility—then you may not receive holiday pay. Generally, you'll still get your normal pay, as per your guaranteed hours.

Paid Time Off (PTO)

What is their policy on accruing PTO hours and are sick days included in those hours or in addition to them?

Sign-on and completion bonuses

Quite often, travel companies will give you a-sign-on bonus (paid at the beginning of the contract) and/or a completion bonus (paid at the end of the contract), as an incentive to get you to sign a contract. Some companies give completion points instead of cash. You can then redeem these through online catalogues.

> Before you get wowed by the offer of a bonus, remember that these bonuses are taxed at a higher rate, sometimes as much as sixty percent. It's usually better to get higher stipends over bonuses.

▸ Length of Contract

Most contracts start at thirteen weeks. If you're not familiar with the facility, it's a good idea to stick with the thirteen-week contract, and then extend if you like it.

Remember to keep track of your weeks worked in the same location, as you must work UNDER twelve months to keep your traveler status. Your recruiter will usually remind you of this and watch for it, but ultimately it's up to you to stay aware. However, as mentioned previously, the recruiter may not realize the government considers a three-month break only a vacation, which means the government may include that break when tallying your time worked.

Also worth repeating—a seven-month break between going back to the same location is an acceptable break to the government, as long as you also have shown no previous plans to return.

CONTINUING YOUR INSURANCE COVERAGE

Your health insurance coverage lasts only as long as your contract, so how will you continue coverage between assignments? Look into COBRA (Consolidated Omnibus Budget Reconciliation Act of 1985). You'll have to pay out-of-pocket, but you'll be covered.

▸ Hours Worked

Often in a contract, it'll state that if the facility gets slow, they can call you off one or two days per pay period. Make sure you are aware of this clause if it's in your contract. If this is a concern for you, ask for a guaranteed forty hours per week.

Get all guaranteed hours written in your contract. Some facilities may only guarantee thirty-five hours a week, while others may guarantee forty.

▸ Time off - Preventing Burnout

If you are expecting to take time off during your assignment, make sure those dates are put into your contract.

To help prevent burnout, vary assignment locations and type of facility in which you'll work. Take time off between assignments or even take a break with a fun seasonal job.

▸ Breaking a Contract

No one expects to break a contract, but sometimes unforeseen things come up for you or for the facility. It's important to check the fine print related to this subject before you sign your contract. Usually there's a one-month notice needed on either end to break a contract, although some locations give only a two-week notice which can be kind of rough. For your peace of mind, ask for a thirty-day notice if possible.

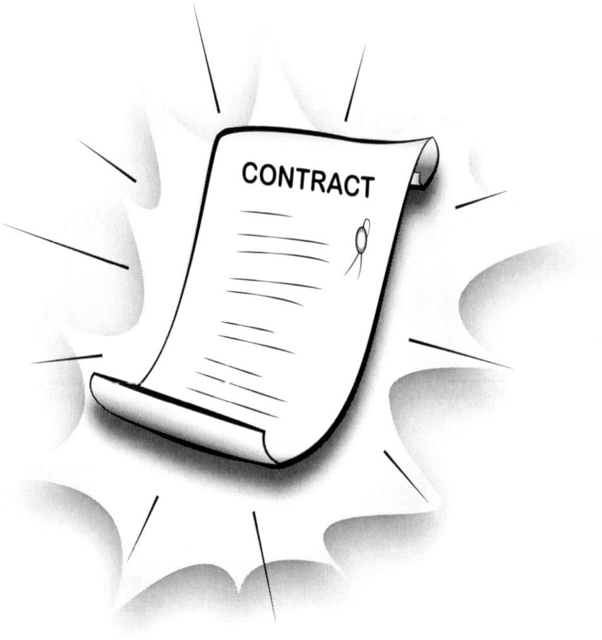

Contracts are rarely broken. That being said, it did actually happen to us on our first assignment, which was very discombobulating to say the least.

On our first assignment, the hospital was having problems and broke our three-month contract after only a month. They did give a one-month notice so all in all the contract was only one month short, but it was enough to send us into newbie panic. Thank goodness we had a supportive recruiter.

Remember, the job is not in the bag until *BOTH* parties sign the contract!

Anything can happen before a contract is signed. Some travelers have interviewed for jobs only to find that a local employee decided to take it. Always keep things in perspective. If it was stressful throughout the process or didn't work out at the last minute, then it's good you didn't take the job and have it backfire on you after a few weeks.

There are so many good assignments, so don't let the one-that-got-away get you down. And don't panic—another one will be right around the corner.

We did tend to panic at the end of each assignment, at least for the first few years. Still, each time after signing on with a new contract, we would realize that everything always worked out so we'd promise ourselves not to panic the next time... We did finally get it. We might still feel the anxiety creeping up but we recover much faster these days.

▸ Checklist

Find out what they offer, negotiate to match your needs, and put in your requests for time off. Have this list with you when talking to your recruiter for each new assignment.

Each assignment contract will be different, so not everything on this list will apply every time.

- ❑ ***Number of facilities in which you'll be working*** – make sure the name of each facility are listed
- ❑ ***Pay***
- ❑ ***Stipends / Per Diems*** – get maximum allowed
- ❑ ***Reimbursements*** – cost of relocation to a new location and/or cost during your assignment for driving between facilities or home health locations (gas and time).
- ❑ ***Bonuses*** – start and/or completion bonuses
- ❑ ***Personal time off (PTO)*** – is sick time calculated separately?
- ❑ ***Holiday Pay***
- ❑ ***Housing*** – negotiate the amount if you'll find your own
- ❑ ***Guaranteed hours per week and call off days/hours***
- ❑ ***Request time off if needed***

Part C

Preparing for Your New Assignment

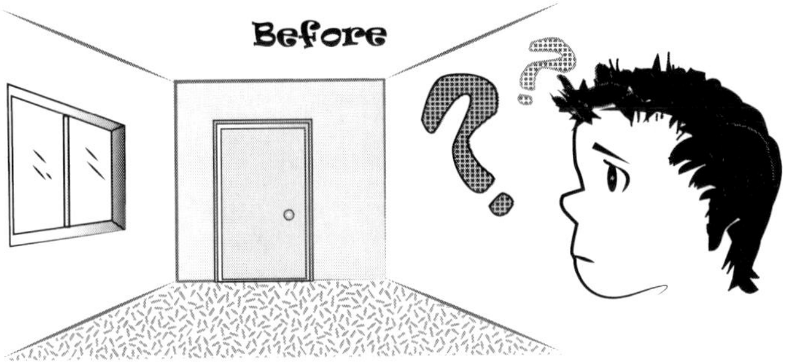

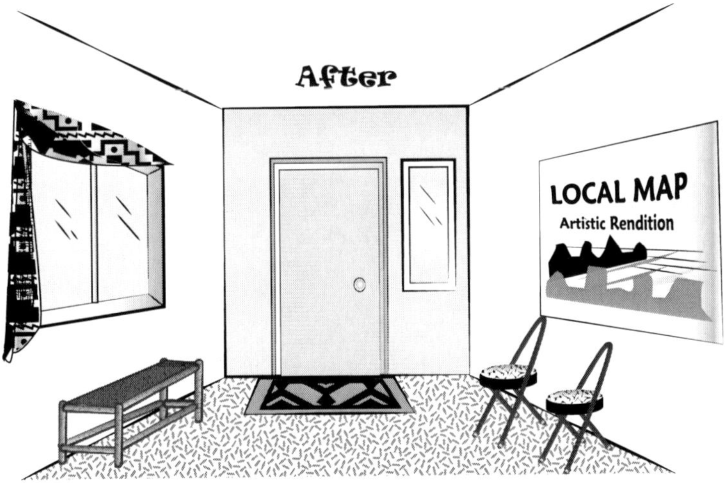

...and creating a temporary home

I'm Official! Now What? 6

Preparing for Your Assignment

- Giving notice
- Mail service
- Vehicle prep
- City and facility research
- Packing
- Pets
- Rental references

New Housing – Who Finds It?

- How to find your new home?
- Applying for a rental, what do you need?

Getting to Your New Location

Setting Up a Home

- Tax service
- Utilities

Staying in Touch with Friends and Family

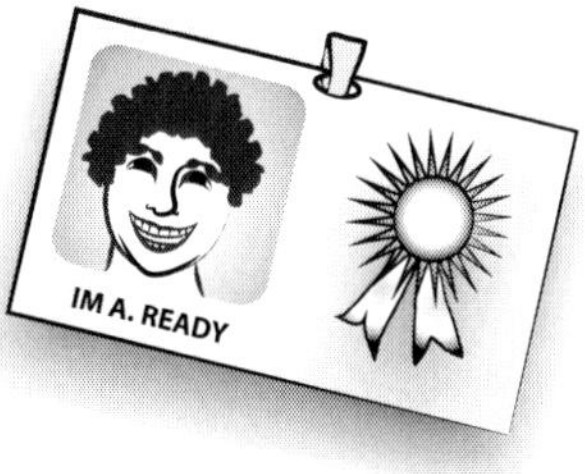

▸ Preparing for Your Assignment

Like I mentioned previously, you can start getting ready for your first assignment a month before—however, I would highly recommend giving yourself two or three months to prepare. You're probably already busy with your full-time job, which leaves little time to take care of the details, phone calls, running around, paperwork, and packing.

Giving notice

Make sure you've given at least a one-month notice to your current landlord if you're renting. Also, make note of the contact person and address of your rental company/individual, as you'll need it for your reference list.

You'll also want to give notice to your current employer as soon as possible so they can find a replacement and you can attain a favorable Letter of Recommendation.

When you give notice to your utility companies, make sure to put their information on your reference list and get an actual letter of reference, if possible. For your future job locations, some utility companies won't charge you a deposit if you have a favorable recommendation of at least one year in good standing, from your previous utility company.

Mail service

If you're getting your mail sent to general delivery at the post office, know where your new, temporary branch is located. You can have your mail delivered directly to you by the Post Office each time you move, but that can cause confusion and crossed wires. A more popular way to deal with your mail is to have it forwarded to you by friends, family, or a mail company. Just remember to have them hold the mail between assignments until you get your new address. Believe me, it's no fun getting your tax papers sent to the wrong address!

We rent a box at a local mail service company in our primary location, then simply have them forward or hold mail as needed.

Vehicle prep

Remember to get your vehicle checked as soon as possible in case any parts need to be ordered for repairs. It's always a good idea to have this taken care of well BEFORE your vehicle is packed and on the road.

Also, make sure your insurance card is up-to-date and that you have the most current one easily accessible.

We once got pulled over for speeding in northeastern Washington, along with a whole row of cars (yes, they can actually do that). To our chagrin, we found that the insurance card in our glove compartment was out-of-date. Luckily, however, we had our important-papers file with accurate insurance card close at hand (only under two piles of stuff). Furthermore, we didn't get a ticket after we told the officer where we were heading to work. He, like everyone else we told, had an odd look on his face and just said, "Good luck."

City/facility research

Know what your new facility is like, what you're expected to wear, and a bit about your new temporary home/city. Your recruiter may have some advice for you, plus it's a good idea to talk to the traveler you'll be replacing. For city information, you can check online sites such as *city-data.com*, chambers of commerce, visitors' bureaus, etc.

Packing

It's helpful to pack as much stuff as you can at least two weeks before you leave, as there'll be lots to do and decisions to be made along the way. Plus, you'll need free time for visits and bon voyage get-togethers with family and friends.

After noting, packing, and sequestering the things you think you'll need, next will come packing for long-term/temporary storage and unloading unwanted stuff to friends, garage sales, or thrift stores.

We packed away a lot into a storage unit on our property and left more generic/general stuff in the house. Over the next two years, every time we came home and wandered through our storage unit, we'd find more things we could let go of. We took stuff to the library, used bookstores, and thrift stores. After realizing how easy it really is to acquire "stuff", we found that whittling our twelve boxes of stored books down to three plus the one we traveled with was easy. (It took us a few years to realize this.)

Okay, now that you've cleared and cleaned your home and have everything you want to travel with in nice little piles by the door, what should you pack it all into?

For a while, we used big rubber storage containers, which were good but too heavy and bulky. Then we went to a thrift store and got lots of rolling suitcases—large ones for light stuff and smaller for heavier—and that worked great.

A friend of ours uses mostly trash bags and duffel bags, which conform to the spaces in her car. So, whatever works for you is great. Just remember you may have to haul your stuff upstairs or across a parking lot. Smaller containers may seem like more hassle, but then again, they may save your back.

For more information on what to pack, see Chapter 10, "What Should I Travel With?"

Pets

We've met travelers with dogs, cats, and rodents. Hopefully, before you've signed a contract, you've already decided which, if any, pets you're going to take and how to transport them. It's a great idea to start crate training as soon as you can before you leave. Not only will this keep your critter safe while traveling and in the new location, but when they feel comfortable in their crate, it'll feel like home no matter where you happen to be.

Our pup puts herself to bed every night in her soft crate no matter where we are.

We've known a few therapists who travel with large dogs. The dogs simply slept their mornings away in their crates, broken up by a nice run at lunch time, and went back into their crates until their after-work run.

Small dogs, especially those still in the chewing and potty training stage, can be placed in a small crate, or you can set them up in a larger wire crate (much like a covered playpen) with a pee pad/ litter box, food and water, and bed.

Once you get to your new location, it's helpful to find a good veterinarian and, if need be, a pet sitter. There may be challenges finding housing that allows pets, but if they're small, even apartments and condos generally allow them, for a fee. One couple, traveling with large dogs, worked around housing issues by traveling with and living in their travel trailer.

After a few years pet free, we now travel with a ten-pound Chihuahua-Italian Greyhound pup adopted from the humane society. We litter box trained her when we were in snow country, as this poor pup didn't have much fur, she did finally enjoy the snow as soon as I knitted her some chaps and a sweater. The great thing about small pets is that they can travel with you, in the cabin, on many airlines as long as they're under a certain weight. When we fly with her, she stays in a backpack carrier stored under our seat. Then during a layover, we simply walk her to the rest room, put down a pee pad, and let her do her business.

Rental references

If you're a renter and plan to find your own housing, remember to get a letter of reference from your landlord as well as from your utility company. If you were in your place for less than a year, get the references from your previous landlord and utility company. You'll need this information when you rent your new home. Most likely, you won't have to have the reference from the utility company, but having it usually means that you don't have to put down a big deposit before turning on your utilities.

If you're a homeowner and renting out or letting family stay at your place, make sure all details are ironed out with your tenants, family, or property management company. Remember that you'll need to maintain a primary residence while you're traveling. If you rent your place out, it may or may not hold up as a primary residence.

▸ New Housing

How to find your new home

There are many ways to go about finding housing. The simplest is to let the travel company find it for you. This may be less of a hassle, but it also leads to less control over where you live.

If you're getting your housing taken care of, then you won't need the following information. You'll just need to research the location, move in, and unpack.

See chapter five under Housing for more information.

For those finding their own housing, always check to make sure the place allows for short-term rental contracts rather than the more common ones of six or twelve months. Many big complexes will allow shorter contracts.

You can look up rentals on *craigslist.org*, online newspapers, and with real estate/property management companies. You can also check out large housing complexes online and see if they offer virtual tours. Also, talk to one of the travelers at the location where you'll be working, especially the one you'll be replacing.

Most of the time we did preliminary research online then committed to a place only after checking it out in person. That way can definitely create headaches and the financial outlay of a hotel stay. However, we always found it was worth it, especially for extended contracts.

It's also important to run any possible rental by locals or the police department.

NEGOTIATE YOUR HOUSING ALLOWANCE

First check to find the going rate for corporate housing in your contracted area, then negotiate with the recruiter for that amount. You will usually need to send rental receipts to your recruiter, as well.

After we negotiated for the housing allowance, we'd look for unfurnished housing and furnish it with what we brought along and sometimes additional items from secondhand stores. If you're good at living simply, you can save a nice amount of money this way. After a few assignments, we made enough for a trip to Ireland.

Housing options

Do you want furnished/unfurnished, roommate/your own place, apartment/condo, cottage/guesthouse, smoking/non-smoking, pet friendly, family friendly? What amenities do you want (laundry, pool, gym)? Do you want a place close to town or rural? What price do you want to pay?

Renting a room in a house will give you someone to connect with. Since the place will probably be furnished, it'll save on the headache of setting up a home. We've had traveler friends who really enjoy this living situation but said it's very important to make sure you feel comfortable with your roommates before moving in.

Still other travelers find it easiest to simply tow their home-on-wheels. Then they only need to find a local travel trailer park.

If you want a nicer and safer rental unit, then go up an extra $100-$200 from the median price. The cost can be worth it, especially when you're not familiar with the area.

We usually look for a place near downtown and the bus stop, since we only bring one vehicle, and we pay the extra few hundred dollars to get a nice, safe place near the facility.

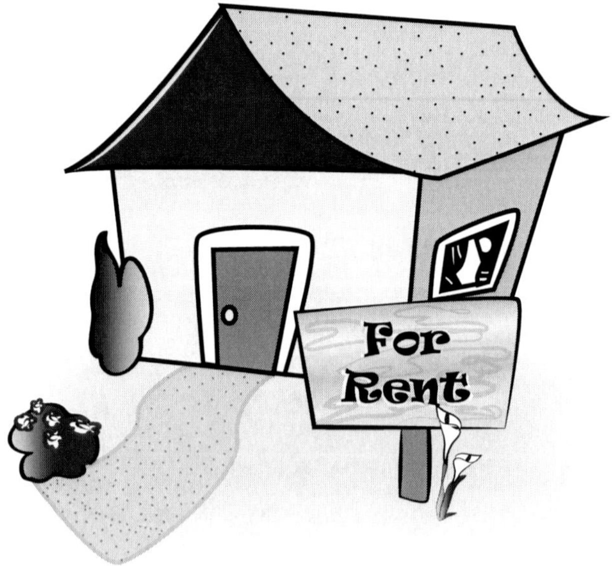

After you've settled into your new home, you'll probably hear other travelers talking about the perfect place they got for less than what you paid. You may also hear about those who are paying double for less than what you have. Either way, hopefully you will already be happy with your own piece of paradise and so can just smile.

Applying for a rental - what do you need?

Each place is different, but most places we rented asked for all or most of the following information. It'll be helpful if you have this all jotted down on one piece of paper, sans your social security card and driver's license number, then just add to it each time you move.

- ❑ ***Name and telephone numbers of past landlords*** (usually for one year), or if you are a homeowner, then the same information for your property management company.
- ❑ ***Employer (Travel company) information*** and length of time with that company
- ❑ ***Name and address of the facility where you'll be working*** including supervisor's name and number
- ❑ ***Vehicle description and license plate number***
- ❑ ***Drivers license number***
- ❑ ***Social Security number***

▸ Getting to Your New Location

When traveling between assignments, have your important papers close at hand, as well as a packed backpack with toiletries and a few changes of clothes. It's frustrating and sometimes embarrassing to have to unload everything in the hotel parking lot to get to your clean socks.

Maps – Plan Route

Make sure to have your car full of gas, your oil checked, and your basic route planned out. Even if you have a GPS, it's good to get a big picture view via a hard copy map in the off chance something happens to your GPS/phone signal. (It's happened to us.)

Get there early to scope out the place

Getting to your location as early as possible will save on mental stress. You'll be able to get moved in and get the lay of the land before jumping into work. No matter when you arrive, it's important to be able to navigate to your new facility before the first day of work.

No matter when you arrive, it's important to be able to navigate to your new facility before the first day of work.

▸ Setting Up a Home

Tax Service

Taxes are dealt with differently for a traveler. You'll need to complete tax forms for EACH state you worked in that year, in addition to completing taxes in your primary location. So, if you're going to have a professional do your taxes for you, it's important to find someone who's familiar with travelers.

You might want to check with your current tax agent to see if you can continue with them by mail. Some tax consultants looked at us strangely when we'd asked if they were familiar with taxes for traveling physical therapists. If we asked them instead if they were familiar with doing taxes for traveling nurses, they could make the leap.

Utilities

If you're renting a place that doesn't come with paid utilities, then find out as soon as possible who to call to get them turned on. In most apartments where the utilities are left on, you'll just need to call to put them in your name. Remember also to get them taken out of your name when you move, to avoid getting billed until someone else moves in. If you get a furnished place, then utilities are usually included. If they are not included, ask your landlord for the names of the local utility companies and get them hooked up right away.

Deposit

Most utility companies charge you a deposit if you don't have a letter of recommendation from your last utility company The letter of recommendation needs to be from the official place where you've made regular payments in good standing for at least a year. You'll still have to pay hookup fees.

It's handy to make copies of the letter of recommendation and keep it in a file with all rental information in order to expedite the process for your following assignments. Make sure, if you gave a deposit, to get it back when you close out.

Phone

Landline: If you'll need dial-up for your computer (rare, these days) or if your family burns through cell phone minutes, then a landline might be a good idea.

Cell Phones: After a lot of careful research, Verizon jumped out as having the best coverage across the country, albeit while being slightly more expensive than the alternatives. We've found this research to be accurate after over five years with them. All that could change at any time, though, so you might want to research further when the time comes.

We also liked that Verizon didn't outsource their customer service department.

Internet Access

Most likely, you'll already have an Internet access company you like. Just make sure it allows national access. Now, how do you get easily changeable Internet hookup? You need dial-up or cable if you go with a landline. You could also simply use your handheld device or tablet that has Internet access or go with a broadband card. These are the choices at present, but stay tuned, as I'm sure this will all continue to get more sophisticated over time.

We started out with a broadband card, although it was pretty slow at that time for streaming. Nowadays we often use our handheld devices. Don't get used to using unsecured Wi-Fi no matter where you are, unless you're not concerned with protecting your information.

Cable/Movies

You can spend the money and get your cable hooked up and travel with your TV or buy a few devices that allow your computer to act like a TV.

We don't have a TV because there are so many interesting things to do in our ever-changing location. Plus, for me, channel surfing is way too addictive. These days, we just watch Netflix.com or Hulu.com. Plus, there are other sites popping up regularly that allow folks to watch TV shows once they've aired.

Many of the broadband cards today have caps on how much you can stream, so DVD rentals are still a plus. There are still some movie rental places around—these gems are fun to peruse and offer more instant gratification than waiting for that DVD to come in the mail. We tend to like old martial arts movies and have been surprised to find amazing collections in the most off-the-wall places. Some folks simply go to their local grocery store to buy or rent movies from the box dispensaries. I tend not to use our credit card at these un-manned video dispensaries, but I know many people who really like the convenience.

Also, don't forget libraries—especially in bigger cities. In Eugene, Oregon, their DVD collection looked like a mini DVD store, and their CD/audio book collections were extensive, as well. Remember, if you're getting a library card, you need to show proof of residence, so bring in your first utility bill.

▶ Staying in Touch with Friends and Family

Today, staying in touch is easy with social networking, cell phones, and email. The important thing to remember, for those not into social networking, is that your friends and family back home are often interested in your adventures (as long as you don't send a three-hour video/slideshow every week). So, dash off an occasional post to let everyone know where you are and how you're doing.

Your New Digs

7

- Checking Out the New Facility
- Your First Day
- Your First Week
- Your First Month

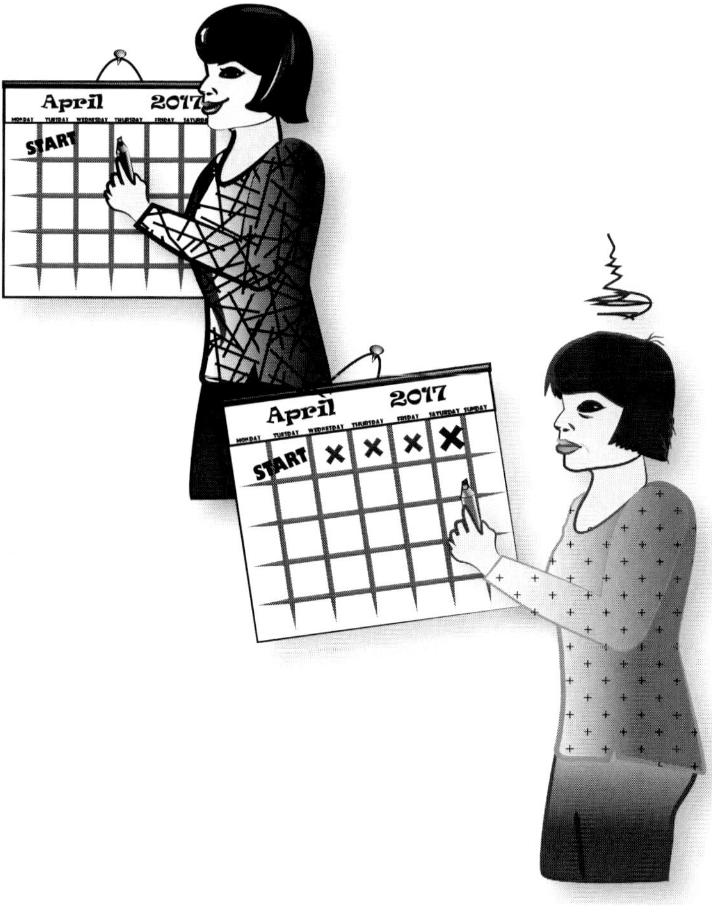

▸ Checking Out the New Facility

You'll want to navigate to the new facility the day before, if not earlier. You can meet the staff and check out the site to get a feel for the place and your coworkers. If you don't already have your housing taken care of, this is a good time to check with locals and other travelers about possibilities. If you're tight on time, then at least just drive to your new facility to get familiar with the route.

▸ Your First Day

What to bring with you?

Bringing your own notepad and clipboard will help you get organized and ready right away. Using a storage clipboard rather than a standard one will allow you to keep your pen, notes, and any cheat sheets handy. Also, pack a lunch and snacks, as you don't know how your day will unfold and what food will be available.

What will likely be expected of you?

For therapists, you'll usually be given a short orientation on how to do your charting, followed by an overview of your case load before hitting the floor. Other therapists will often be around to help you along the way. On some occasions, where most of the staff are newbie travelers, you may not have much help.

Nurses will also have an orientation then will most likely spend the day working with and observing other nurses. Some facilities may require a half- or full-day orientation the first day. If you'll be using an unfamiliar computer charting system, give yourself at least an hour to familiarize yourself.

Pay attention, open your eyes and ears, and ask important questions. You'll find the balance between stepping back and learning and jumping in with confidence.

▸ Your First Week

You'll probably feel tired, under the weather, or a bit off during your first week. This is to be expected. You might be prone to eat more junk food, take more naps, and/or stay home rather than explore your surroundings. You might also have some trouble sleeping at night. Not to worry—you're probably not experiencing a rare brain flu. It's simply your system adjusting to a new location and job routine.

Remember, your brain is taking in new policies, dynamics, patients, and time schedules, so respect the adjustment period.

Also, there's the possibility that the flora may affect you differently, either better or worse. A word to the wise—sticking to any regimens you currently have will help keep you grounded.

Some folks don't have any problems with allergies or altitude adjustments when on vacation, yet under the stress of starting a new job, the body doesn't have as much flexibility, so you may experience more challenges. After your body adjusts, you'll be craving all the new, fun experiences awaiting you in your new location.

In almost every place we've worked, folks have told us that they have the worst allergy season of anywhere. If we felt fine, they'd predict worse problems for us the following year. Take it all with a grain of salt and just listen to your body.

▸ Your First Month

After your first month, you should be feeling pretty grounded in your new job. However, give yourself more adjustment time if this is your first assignment, as you'll probably be continuing to process this career change, in addition to wrapping up things from your primary residence.

Overall, you should now be feeling more energized and curious to start investigating your surroundings and ferreting out all the local gems awaiting you.

If you've recently gone from sea level to higher elevations, be prepared for additional adjustment time. It'll take a while for your body to produce more red blood cells to process the oxygen out of the thinner air.

The more time you take off between assignments, the more time it may take to get refocused and grounded again.

Going from near sea level, at Santa Barbara County, up to 7,000-plus feet at Santa Fe, New Mexico, we both found ourselves more winded than normal, especially on the stairs. Peter also experienced strong altitude-induced vertigo, finally gaining relief with Brandt-Daroff exercises. Once, a family member drove 15 hours straight from Santa Barbara County to visit us. Upon his arrival, we whisked his tired self up to the beautiful Santa Fe ski area, about 10,000-plus feet high. Needless to say, he got very sick, and that's when we learned that the local oxygen bar can be a necessity, not just a spa treatment.

Getting the Lay of the Land - Fun Stuff

8

- People You'll Meet
- Season and Climate Changes
- Getting Around
- Tourist Attractions

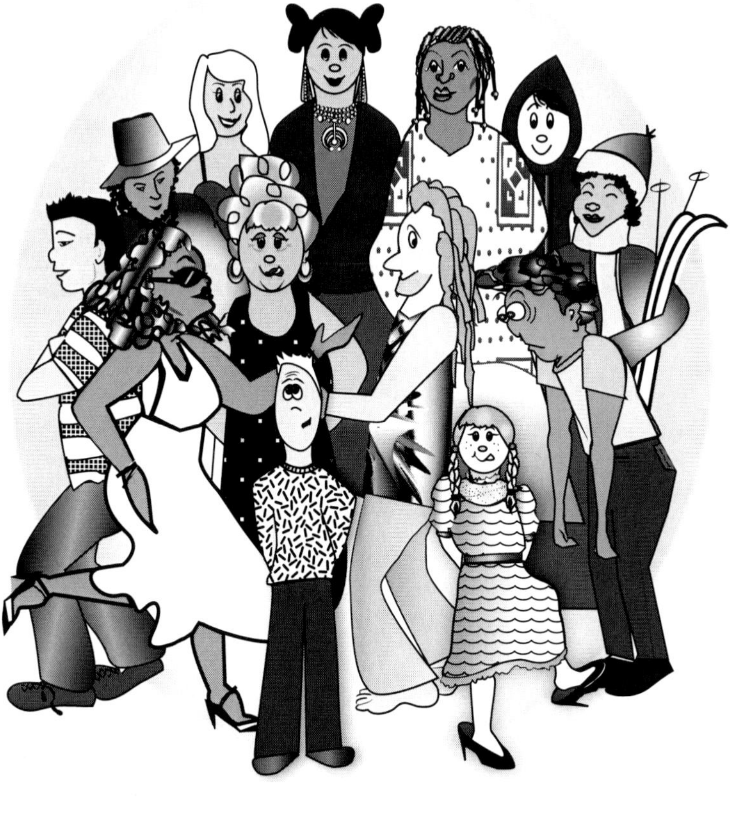

▸ People You'll Meet

One of the most wonderful aspects of this career is interacting with new people and learning about the rich tapestry of cultures we have in our own country. Our own state of California is made up of four very distinct areas/subcultures (north, central coast, central valley, south).

When you realize how similar we all are, you can style flex and have fun at the Country Music Catfish Fry—watch out for those aggressive elderly ladies toting their own bottles of catsup; they have sharp elbows!—or sway to the music with dread-headed locals at an outdoor world music festival. Just don't breathe in too deeply, or things will starting getting a bit surreal. If the trees start walking around, take a break and inhale some fresh air.

Everywhere you go, there'll be different cultures and subcultures. The one thing we found that remains the same from the hippie areas of northern California to the gun-friendly Texans is that most people want exactly the same thing: peace of mind and a good life for themselves and their children.

In the Texas hill country, we were surprised to find that cowboy hats gave way to caps, as this is predominantly an orchard farming area rather than a cattle ranching one. And we were doubly surprised to find the predominant subculture was German.

In Washington, we drove a short ways from the dynamic city energy of drizzly Seattle to quiet, dry, and sunny Sequim. There, locals invited us to a salmon fry. Only a few hours away, we found ourselves in Forks, a temperate rain forest! The subcultures in each area seem to change subtly with the changes in predominant weather and terrain.

▸ Season and Climate Changes

If you go from a rainy or humid climate to a dry area (or vice versa), relative to where you were last, give your system a bit of time to make that adjustment.

Remember the importance of moisturizing and hydrating in hot dry climates, as well as the importance of staying out of the intense noon sun. If you're going to a drier area, you might experience nosebleeds, headaches, and ringing in your ears. An old Ayurvedic regime is to use salve, olive oil, or castor oil to protect ears and nose in dry weather and in cold areas with dry heat.

In cold climates, you'll want good nonslip shoes, and don't forget the secrets to staying warm: thermals, hats, and scarves. Make sure your vehicle is in good working order and that you have good tires, chains, and emergency supplies in case you get stranded.

When we first came to experience snow country—after years in moderate climate lowlands—I slipped twice on black ice and sprained an ankle due to ink-black skies and uneven surfaces. Peter almost got lost after getting turned around on a snow hike, and we once narrowly missed getting stuck in a snowstorm with the rest of the traffic on Interstate 80. We eventually learned to be prepared.

▸ Getting Around

GPS/Maps

So what's better—using your Global Positioning Sevice (GPS) device, or hitting up the local AAA? We got a GPS in our second year of traveling, and it cut down on our stress, especially in larger cities. It did often send us to the wrong side of the street and occasionally to the middle of nowhere. Our new GPS is vastly improved. We still hit up AAA and cross-reference things with online maps, but the GPS is nice, especially if you're alone in the car. Making sure your GPS is updated saves a lot of headaches.

We now mostly use the GPS on our phones but do reference the old TomTom GPS, as well as paper maps since we've had our phones lose signal at the most inopportune times.

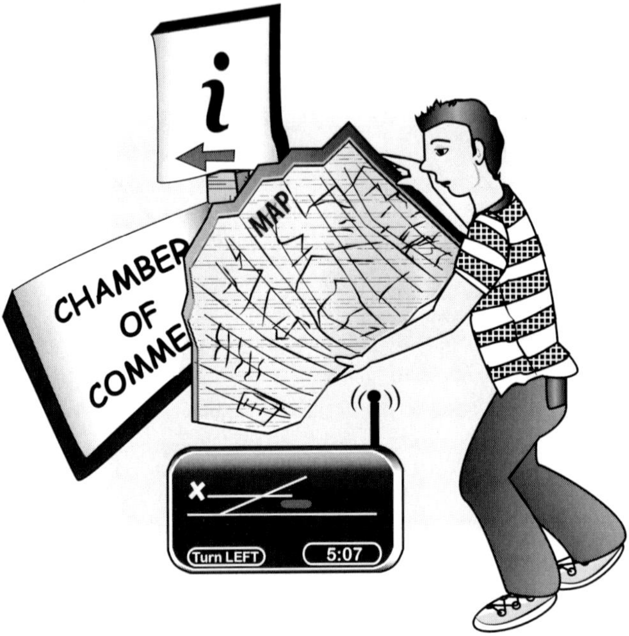

The local phone book

Keep this handy reference on hand, since sometimes it's quicker than your smartphone. You can look up what you want, then input the address into the GPS—again, especially handy if you have a problem with your phone's power or signal.

Chamber of commerce and newspapers

You'll want to check out the helpful folks at the local chamber of commerce. Sometimes they're also combined with a tourist and visitors' bureau, so you can get information about moving to their community, plus information on touristy things to do. They usually have phone books as well, so grab one for the house and one for the car.

More good places to find out about your location are the local newspapers and weekly arts and entertainment tabloids. Most larger newspapers have an Arts & Entertainment section at least once a week. Tourist cities often have a special magazine or journal for local events.

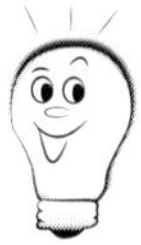

In order to keep from being bogged down with paper 'stuff,' gather all you've collected (pamphlets, journals, papers, and fliers), mark compelling events on your calendar, then cut out and staple together interesting tidbits or tape then to the calendar. Recycle the rest.

▸ Tourist Attractions

If you want to save money on tourist attractions, then before you visit, check to see if they have specials for residents. Some museums and galleries have certain free nights and/or specials for locals. Some places will give you a discount if you show a local library card or utility bill with your picture ID. Others want to see a local driver's license. Since your time in each location is only temporary, explore the area for all the interesting things it has to offer.

Community Events

Check out the calendar of events on multiple local tourism web-sites and in local newspapers and magazines. Often sites and publications will list events differing from each other, so check around. Some communities are supportive of poster boards, so ferret out these along sidewalks, in coffee shops, at pubs, or anywhere people gather. You can even look up your location on Facebook.com and meetup.com to see what comes up.

Library

We saved a lot of money when we spent time at the local libraries. Many libraries have a good selection of things to entertain and enlighten, as well as information and fliers of local happenings. Even the smaller libraries often have a used book sales area.

In Eugene, Oregon, *we took full advantage of their wonderfully huge library—it turned into a weekend destinations spot. Besides 'readables', it also housed a computer lab, a used bookstore, a coffee shop, and a huge selection of DVDs and CDs. We would spend hours perusing the 'readables', audios, 'watchables', and interesting happenings posted on their bulletin board, all whilst sipping cappuccinos.*

In the charming town of Silver City, New Mexcio, we would walk the two blocks to the little library and peruse the 'readables'. When we found something interesting on the sale shelf, we'd simply drop our money into the donation can.

Old Town

Many communities have a designated old town, full of history and charming shops. Every community has a history, and usually information can be found on plaques sprinkled about, discovered at the museum, or just viewed in the old dilapidated buildings. Your trip into old town will be much enhanced if you do some community research first.

Physical Activities and Adventures

Here you'll again get information from all the channels listed above as well as from the city's parks and recreation department and the county and state parks' departments.

Remember to pick the brains of the locals for local hot spots, although you'll want to continue to research and explore above and beyond their ideas. We often discovered places the locals had either never heard of or had forgotten about. It's kind of like us growing up in California and not visiting Yosemite.

In each place we land, we spend a lot of time exploring local hiking and walking trails and camping areas. In Eugene, Oregon, we were thrilled with their network of bike trails. In New Mexico, we could never get enough of exploring the ruins, powdery snow, and beautiful scenery. And throughout each job, we usually spent time hunting up local disc golf courses.

Night Life

In most areas, you'll find interesting places such as eateries, performing arts venues, nightclubs, pubs, coffee shops, and bookstores. Some areas, usually the larger cities, offer opera and Broadway performances, as well. Search out (via phone book, brochures, advertisement, internet, word of mouth, etc.) places you're drawn to and see what they offer.

Shopping

We noticed when in central Texas that the community was incorporated if there was a waterway, a place of worship, a Sonic and/or Dairy Queen, and a Walmart. Not much more was needed by the locals, and sometimes there wasn't much more offered. In cases like this, we found we enjoyed living simply, and we just made it an adventure to occasionally travel to a bigger city to forage. Sometimes we resorted to ordering online, but more often than not, it was more fun to hunt for it locally and support the local economy.

Thrift/Consignment Stores

Don't underestimate these humble treasure troves. In some bigger cities, we found huge thrift stores with their own used bookstores and loads of antiques from Europe, plus the humbler stuff like clothes and home furnishings. Many now even have a section of brand-new items.

Thrift stores can also be a big help if you don't own snow clothing and winter is fast approaching—you can even find skis. It's also nice to visit a thrift store for those things you left behind (wine glasses, pans, bike helmets, lamps, etc.) or temporary furniture like a chair or a coffee table, which you can then re-donate when your assignment is over. If you want to go a step up, then check out the consignment and retro stores. They often carry higher quality merchandise.

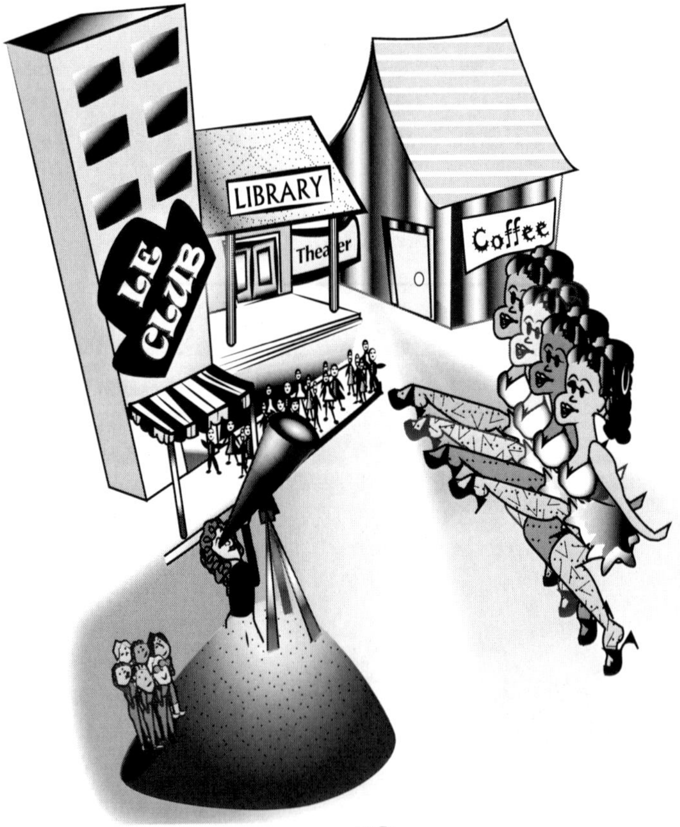

Part D
Packing Up & Moving Out

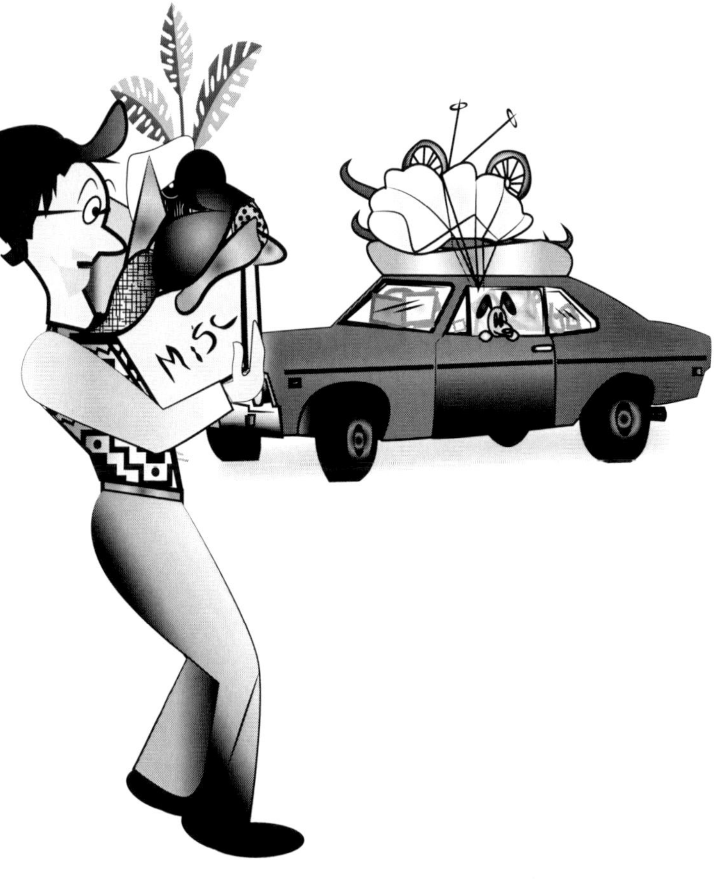

Your first & successive assignments

What Should You Pack? 9

- What Should You Travel With?
- General Tips
- Creating a Homey Feeling
- Helpful Electronic Doodads
- Collecting While on the Road

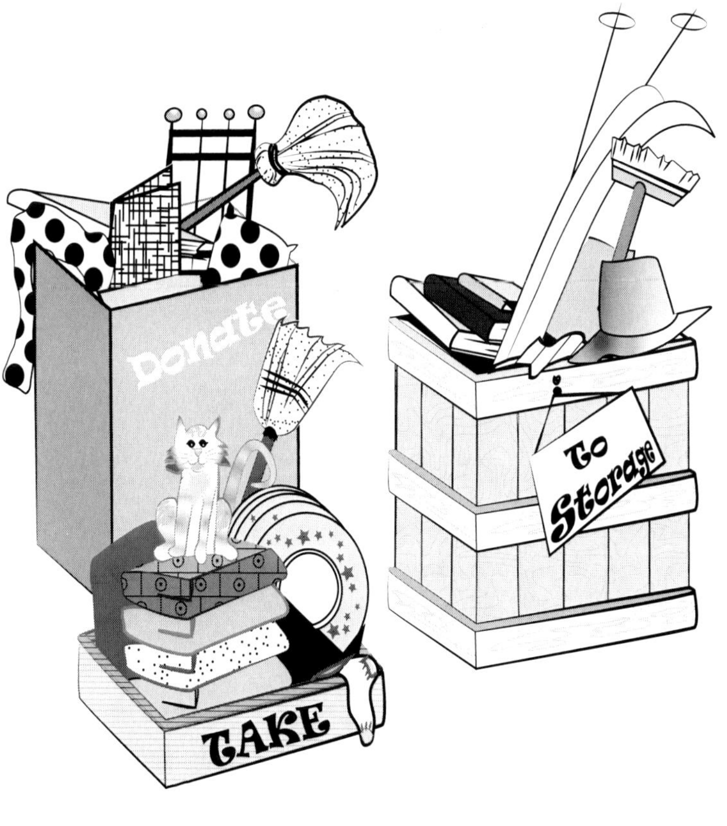

▸ What Should You Travel With?

First, you'll have to figure out if you want a furnished or unfurnished place, or simply to take your fully stocked home with you in a travel trailer. If you're going for a furnished place, then you probably won't need much beyond your personal items, toys, and special cooking supplies.

This chapter is a compilation of what you might need for a furnished place, plus all the extras you'll need if it's unfurnished.

The strange thing is, even if you pack everything you think you'll need, you'll still find yourself bringing in more bags of "stuff" over the course of your assignment, so pack lightly but well.

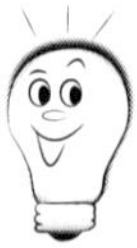

* Take items that have more than one use.

* Use packing containers that can be used for décor and/or furniture (wicker laundry basket, wooden box for coffee table, etc.)

* Look for nice, sturdy folding furniture (collapsible book case, folding bench/table, wire baker's rack, etc.)

* Use cloth scarves, tapestries, cloth napkins, towels, and place mats as packing material, then repurpose as wall art and clothing accessories (the scarves, not the napkins!).

We've heard interesting stories about what some therapists like to travel with—from their special loveseat and tap dance boards to their favorite gerbils.

We always travel with a plethora of musical instruments—including a full-size digital piano—paint and knitting supplies, bikes, camping gear, and favorite books. Yes, we used to get it all into our little van, but these days we use a rooftop soft pack along with our bike rack.

Everyone has special items they like to travel with, but here I want to cover some of the more mundane things that you may not realize you'll need.

Bathroom

* Keep a well-stocked, accessible first aid kit.

* A washable shower curtain, easy on/off hooks, and a rug will make your place feel more homey.

* Dr. Bronner's liquid castile soap is good to have on hand. In a pinch it can be used for detergent, shaving cream, soap, and household cleaner.

* Don't forget the shavers, tweezers, scissors, lotion, sunscreen, bug repellent, and the like.

Always have a roll of toilet tissue with you, as most unfurnished places won't have any. This can be an unpleasant surprise.

* A temporary trash can might be found at a local thrift store or just hang a plastic bag on the toilet paper holder.

* Bring or buy a small toilet brush and plunger.

* Décor ideas: Use the fancy mugs you've collected to hold your toothpaste and toothbrush. A flat basket hung on the wall, with a few paperclips added for hooks, will artfully

display your jewelry and be easy to pack away. Wrap it in a towel then later just unwrap it and hang it.

Tools

* Bring some sturdy, basic tools for your car, like a jack, electrical tape, pliers, a wrench, and a cutting implement.

* You'll also want to bring a hammer, a Swiss Army knife and/or a multi-ended screwdriver, and duct tape. Why the duct tape? Well, who knows, but you can use it for just about anything.

Kitchen

* **Cooking supplies**

  We enjoy cooking yet still only need one large cast iron skillet (can use it also for baking), large cooking pot, sauce-pan, glass square baking pan with lid (doubles as a storage dish), and a cookie sheet or two.

Remember, all ovens will be slightly different, and baking times will need to be adjusted for higher altitudes. Watch out for those charming old-fashioned stoves. Although they're fun to look at, they can be very temperamental.

Once on assignment, we got blown against the wall while trying to light one for the umpteenth time.

Don't forget the spatulas (wooden, metal, rubber), ladle, a quality can/ bottle opener, grater, measuring cup, and measuring spoons.

Slow cookers can be helpful, and some people even bring a mini microwave, coffee maker, toaster (though if you're watchful, you can use the broiler for toast), blender, electric mixer, and fruit juice squeezer. It's best to use compact but sturdy brands that will travel well. We tend just to bring a French press and our Vitamix blender.

* Eating supplies

We bring two sturdy camping plates, two stoneware plates (stoneware holds up well and can be heated in the oven), a few oversized bowls that can be used for soups or for mixing bowls.

A few ceramic and travel mugs, and possibly a couple of wine glasses should do you fine. If you need additional glasses or cups and don't want to haul them, you can get them for pennies as you go.

A large sharp knife and a few steak and butter knives, spoons, and forks should be enough—but again, they're pretty inexpensive if you feel you need more on the road.

* Storage containers

Most likely you'll accidentally start accumulating containers when you buy groceries. Still, if you do find you need something specific, then get the stacking freezer safe containers as they'll nest easily for packing, and you'll be able to freeze extras.

Remember that you'll need to make your artwork usable (again with the usable art theme!). So collecting colorful tins is a great way to store your teas, big utensils, and whatnots to create a homey/tidy atmosphere. When moving, you can use these containers to pack sensitive items, or in the case of baggies of teas and spices, just put the lid on, and you're ready to go. Make sure the bags are sealed well since garlicky cinnamon and minty curry may not be the flavors you want to encourage.

*** Cloth Supplies**

Cloth napkins, dish towels, and a kitchen floor runner won't just look nice but will have other uses as well. The cloth napkins and dish towels can be used as packing material when en route, and if they're cotton, they can be used as pot holders. The kitchen runner will help catch spills, which will aid your ability to recoup your cleaning deposit with less work.

*** Cleaning Supplies**

You'll want to buy or bring along some nontoxic cleaners that have multiple uses, such as white vinegar (window cleaning, paint removal, unclogging drains, fabric softener, floor cleaner, etc.), Citra Solv, BonAmi, baking soda (teeth, jewelry, cooking, with vinegar to unclog drains), dish detergent, and Dr. Bronner's liquid soap.

Not only is nontoxic better for you and the environment, but you'll also be happy it's nontoxic if it accidentally tips over while you're traveling (voice of experience). For extra security, secure lids and openings with duct tape (aha! found a use for it already!) Bring a broom, dustpan, mop, and compact vacuum cleaner.

***Food**

Unless you have some specific allergies or needs, you can buy most things when you arrive at your location. Packing some things like spices (take only what you'll really use), baking goods, munchies, and quick foods for your first night will really come in handy.

Also, if you like specialty foods (we love our smoked oysters in olive oil) that can only be found in the big city or in a specific store, fill up on them before leaving for an off-the-beaten-track location. A few of your special items will make you feel more at home in your new location.

Bedroom

We started out with an Aerobed inflatable bed. With an egg crate cushion on top, it was most comfortable, although the egg crate material can sometimes over-heating in hot climates.

We rigorously researched inflatable beds. Aerobed seemed to be a top contender but it still ended up getting leaks that we couldn't find to patch. After a while, we found that a few extra thick camping cushions or a child's bunk bed mattresses worked just as well.

A few sheets, pillows and cases, extra wool blankets, and a down comforter are all we need to be comfortable in any location. Plus, in the van, we keep a few sleeping bags and a blow-up mattress for guests and for camping.

Some secondhand stores sell new and sanitized previous-ly-owned mattresses. It's hard to find mattresses in most thrift stores, as only certain ones, like Salvation Army, have sanitizing machines.

▸ General Tips

* Check the weather before you leave to figure out what you'll need to have on hand along the way to your destination.

  Once, after a quick vacation, we flew from seventy-one degrees Houston, Texas, to twenty-eight degrees Santa Fe, New Mexico. Needless to say, we were very cold while waiting for the plane to taxi in. At the luggage pickup we quickly tore through our possessions to find warm clothes before leaving the airport.

* Pack toiletries like shampoo and conditioner and moist face/body wipes, especially if you'll be camping along the way.

* Baby or foot powder for your sandals or sock-less shoes is important if you're heading to a hot or humid climate.
* If you have long hair, go with hair doodads that are soft. Firm clips can prevent you from fully leaning back in your seat, causing neck pain. Even a minor thing like this can have an effect after a long trip.

▸ Creating a Homey Feeling

Kitchen

Adding a runner, tins, and colorful dishcloths will create a usable and nice touch. Also, since you'll probably want mementos of places you've been, magnets are easy and portable. These collectibles don't take up much room and create an artistic mosaic on the refrigerator, with pictures of friends and family.

Living Areas

Besides our books and hobby items like musical instruments and art supplies, we also bring folding furnishings. We have a slim folding bamboo piece that can be used as a table, bench, and/or computer workstation.

A bamboo bookcase and a metal baker's rack both fold down flat yet look substantial when set up. And they give the room a personal feel.

We've been experimenting with folding chairs, from round to square, but so far haven't found the ultimate one, so we continue to use some classy camping chairs. Also, we bring lots of large floor pillows which work as seats, backrests, extra padding on chairs—and which are helpful as packing material.

After unpacking, we're always left with storage containers to deal with, so we have a few nice ones we leave out and use for everyday stuff like laundry (large basket), magazines (small square

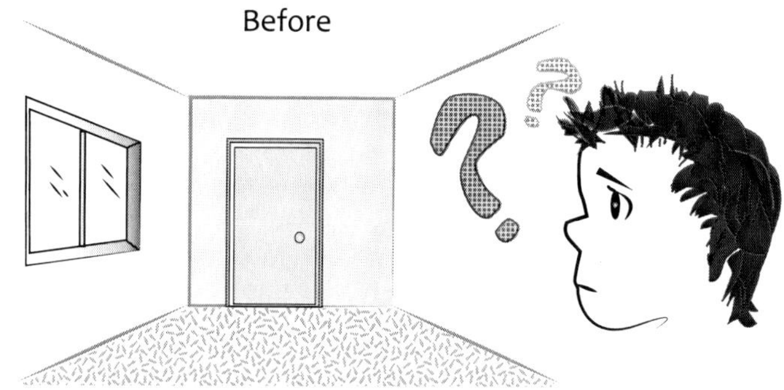

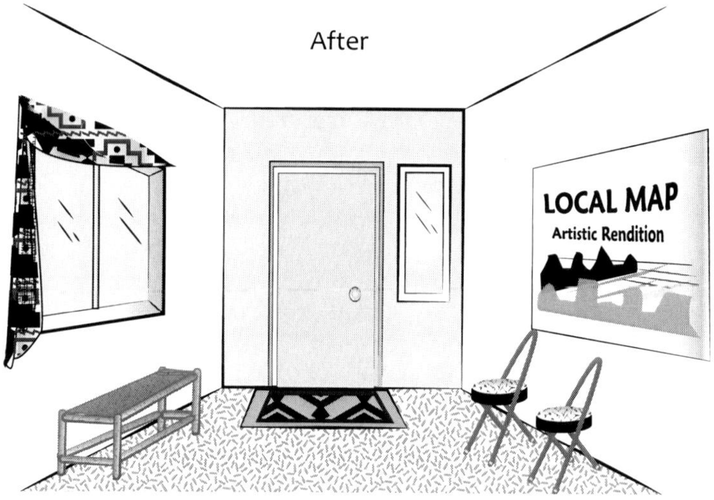

basket), office supplies (colorful child-sized rolling suitcase), etc. Our small bamboo file box gives a bit of cultural ambiance and keeps all our files accessible. The other storage containers, plastic boxes, and soft suitcases simply stack inside each other.

Nice scarves, fabrics, towels, placemats, and tapestries add a sense of comfort to your area,when draped over the door, windows, or hung on walls. When moving, they can be used to wrap around fragile items.

Office

A colorful, child-sized rolling suitcase works great to hold office supplies (office on wheels). Add to it a stapler, scissors, pens, paper clips, pushpins, glue, tape, computer paper and ink, etc.

It's helpful to get a zipping binder to keep all of your bills, checks, important papers, phone numbers, etc. This way, you can keep it all together and near you when you're traveling between assignments. Also, a small portable file box will keep all filed neatly.

▸ Helpful Electronic Doodads

Computer and Speakers

Portable computers are a must. Not only can you use them for traditional computing, but you can also use them for watching movies, storing photos, and storing/listening to your music. You might also want to consider a computer/monitor with a special screen for clearer movie viewing.

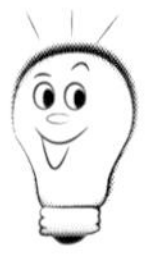

Backup your computer often, either off site or to an external drive. With all your moving, there is a greater chance of breaking the computer or even losing it.

Make sure you get a setup that's powerful enough to do what you want. These days, we don't need as much hard drive space, for we have the option of storing files to an external server (cloud storage). But if you have complicated software, are gaming, or need a lot of storage space, you might want to go with the larger hard drive and RAM capacity.

After three years, we finally got some nice computer speakers through our company's rewards program. What a difference they make!

Internet Wireless Access Card

Back in the early days, this puppy was amazing as it was the only 'affordable' way to access the Internet when out and about and in rural areas. These days, most Personal Digital Assistant (PDAs), iPads, and smartphones allow you this access. The drawbacks at that time were that the wireless access card didn't stream well and might not work as well in certain parts of the house, although I'm sure they're continuing to get better and better. Who knows, maybe by print time, we'll just be uploading and downloading from the Internet directly into our brains! Ha! You laugh now, but just wait!

GPS

A Global Positioning System (GPS) device isn't necessary, but it sure can be helpful, especially when you're alone. It'll usually lead you directly to where you want to go, and often in a calm unhurried voice. (Not so, your copilot after a long day.) Keeping a local phone book in the car will help if you run into any problems.

We didn't have GPS for the first two years we traveled, and we didn't do so badly, but we did get lost and frustrated more often.

These days, we usually use the GPS on our phones, although due to issues with phone access in some areas, we've had to rely on the GPS in our vehicle or an actual hardcopy map (gasp!) on more than a few occasions .

Cell Phone

Cell phones used to be an added assistance but now they seem to be a necessity. You can get affordable family share plans in which phoning between family members are free. You may want to increase your minutes between assignments, as you'll probably be doing a lot of calling outside of your family plan.

We researched the cell phone companies to find out who had the best coverage over the US. Hands down, we found Verizon to be the best for coverage. Other travelers have also concurred. Yet, since things in the cyber world are changing so fast, things might have changed by the time this book comes out. So you'll want to do your own research.

Music playing device

Finally we got an MP3. It's nice, as one of us can use that and the other the computer. Although now we pretty much just use our smartphones to stream music. Some folks use their tablets for music, which they either stream or store on their devices.

Printer with Scanner

You'll want a printer with a scanner so you can quickly scan and email documents to your company. Originally, we got a small, cheap printer that packed easily but stressed out our computer due to all its hidden bloatware. Bloatware is all the extra stuff added to your computer when you install the software unless you're savvy enough to block it. Be aware, the cheapest printers often make up for the low cost with adware (advertisement bloatware) and more expensive ink. Today you can get small all-in-one computers for a decent price. For best deals, just check the reviews and cost per page.

Digital Camera

Our camera feels like a necessity to us, because we like to capture all the amazing places we've been. Most PDAs and cell phones take decent photos, but we usually want the control we get with our mid-priced camera and changeable lenses. We use our photos for social networking with friends and family, as well as for reference material for my paintings.

▸ Collecting While on the Road

Fun and compact items to collect on your travels are postcards, magnets (turn the fridge door into a travelogue album), and mugs (use as drinking containers as well as toothbrush and pen holders). Fun local maps rendered by a local artist are nice for reference and can hang on the wall yet another piece of usable art. We've also collected a few needed coasters.

One traveler hunted up great antiques finds while on her assignments. She'd then shipped them home for storage. Others collect retro clothing, jewelry and pottery made by local tribes, artwork, T-shirts, maps, etc.

I've often been reminded that if you really want an item, then get it, because you might not be back to that part of the country again. But also remember you may be traveling with the items you collect, so make sure you have room for them!

Once, while on assignment in Texas, I went into the music store where Peter had been shopping. As I walked closer to him, the employees began to unconsciously close ranks around him. It was then that I found out he'd bought a full-sized digital piano. I'm not sure if the employees were trying to protect Peter or the piano. Either way they both came away unscathed, but we did have a laugh when it came time to pack at the end the assignment. The piano became our regular traveling companion.

Expediting the Move-Out Process 10

- Prepare from the Beginning
- Cleaning Tips
- Paperwork
- Repacking

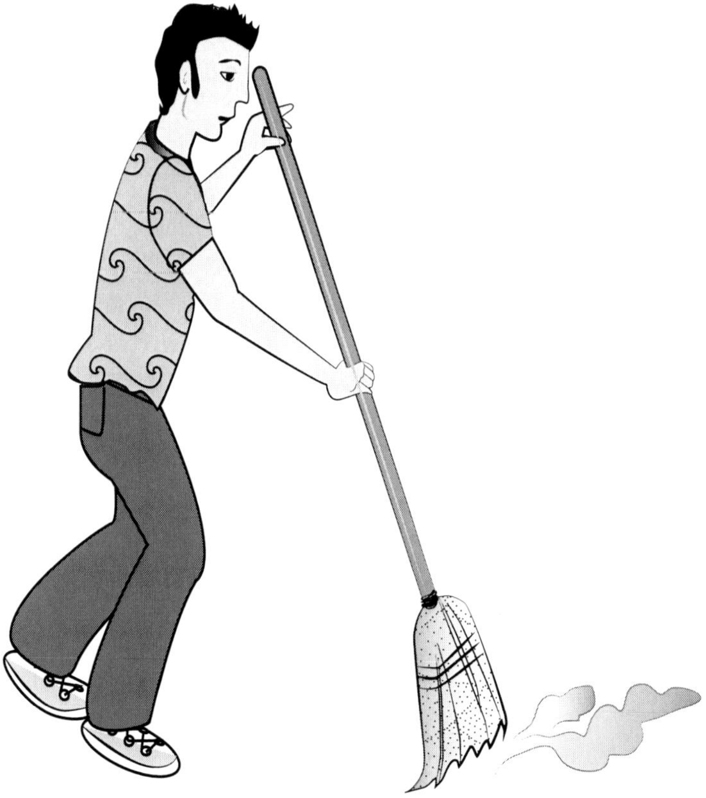

▸ Prepare from the Beginning

Make your move-out process easier by planning for it when you move in.

Put foil over the range's drip pans.

Put an old cookie sheet in the oven to catch drips, although it is said this may cause your food to cook unevenly.

Keep your spices, flavor packets, and hot pepper flakes (from your pizza orders) in one of your colorful tins so the cupboard doesn't get full of powdery residue. When you're ready to move on, you'll only have to tighten the lid, and you're good to go.

Cleaning Tips

If you don't have a self-cleaning oven, then make extra sure you clean any spills right when they happen. A baked-on spill means a lot more elbow grease will be needed to clean it later.

Keeping the baseboards vacuumed or dusted will save on having to scrub them when you move out, especially bathroom and kitchen baseboards, due to moisture mixing with dust.

Do a thorough, whole-house cleaning the week before you leave. Then you'll only have to do a quick once-over when you're down to the wire.

Make sure your pets are litter box, pee pad, or outdoor potty trained as soon as possible. Clean up any critter accidents as soon as they happen, preferably with a smell-neutralizing formula.

▸ Paperwork

Before moving onto your next assignment, you'll want to get a letter of reference from your landlord and your utility company.

Make sure you always update your rental contact information sheet at the end of your contract. If you don't already have one made up, make one while the information is fresh in your mind. This sheet should have all your contact information from your current rental and utility companies and be easily accessible so it's at your fingertips when you find your next place.

It's always less frustrating, in the long run, to update paperwork as you go rather than having to search for the information at a later date.

▸ Repacking

After repacking and before loading up make sure all of your important papers—including contact information and directions for your next assignment—are front and center. You'll want to place this file folder/zippered binder in an easily accessible area, in your vehicle, before you head out. By now you should be getting the idea of just how helpful it is to have all your paperwork prepared and accessible.

Plan to do much of your main packing the week before, for there'll always be more than enough to do right before you leave.

If you've collected a lot on your present assignment, you'll need to get creative to pack it all in. You might even want to invest in an auto rooftop rack and storage unit—a soft rooftop storage unit is easy to stow away when not in use. If you'll still need more space, plan to get a hitch put on your vehicle and rent a moving trailer. Sometimes it takes extra time to order the appropriate hitch, so plan early.

Just before you leave, make sure you have your overnight case accessible and a bag packed with road trip essentials, munchies, and drinks.

Part E
Fun Stuff from the Road

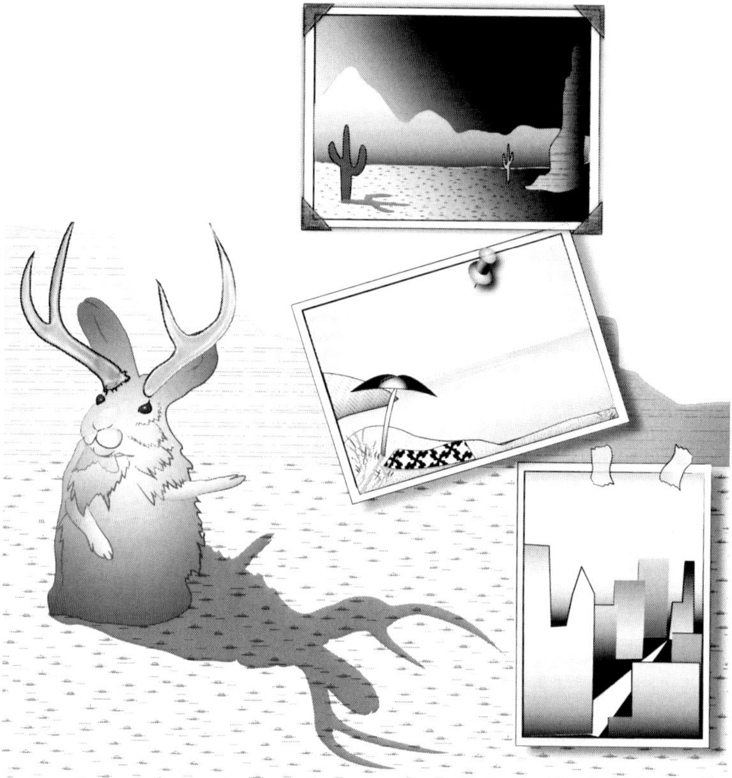

Travelog

11

▸ **Places Worked & Traveled on Assignment**

▸ **Fun Places Traveled between Assignments**

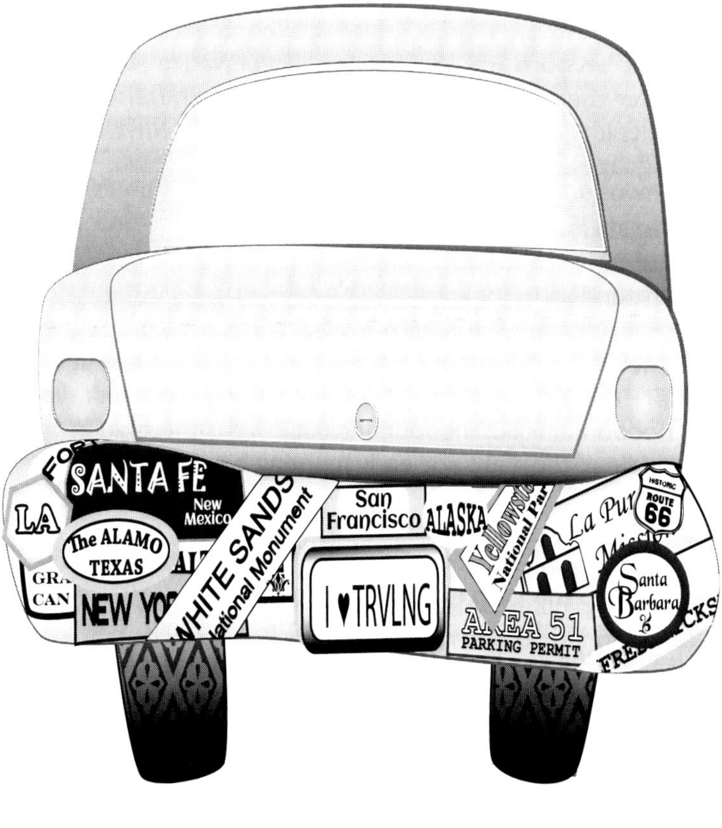

see the mining car that took the men a mile underground. Plus, you'll see an interactive layout of the mining tunnels that run under the community. There is also a refined English Cotswold style home/mansion and gardens where the owner of the mine lived. This area is an artist's dream when lit up in fall colors, snow covered, or full of spring flowers. Don't miss a walk under the climbing roses, and view hundreds of old cultivators in the rose gardens.

On the backside of the mine, enjoy hiking, biking, and horse trails. The trails suit a fast-paced hike or a leisurely stroll.

Hwy 49

Just about anywhere you drive up the 49 from Nevada City, you'll find something that draws you to stop the car. It might be a desire for a hike along the wheelchair-accessible Independence Trail, a dip in the boulder-laden Yuba River, a snowball fight, or a stroll through any number of charming little old towns. After fifteen years, we can still find more to explore.

Center for the Arts

This center has been growing and growing over the years. They attract talent from the San Francisco Bay area, as well as from across the country.

Nevada Theatre, Miner's Foundry, and Off Broad Street Theater

This community takes the cake, with Off Broad Street's live cabaret dessert theater, the historic Nevada Theater with its movies and live plays, and the Miner's Foundry, a happening community hub.

Old Towns of both Communities

You know you've got something special when locals and

tourists alike hang out in the same places. Old town is full of well-priced stores, coffee shops, and some amazing bookstores including the two huge used bookstores in Grass Valley's Old Town. Our favorite coffee shop-used bookstore-dance studio (Tomes/Sierra Mountain Coffee Roasters) is located just between Grass Valley and Nevada City, in the area known as the Brunswick basin.

Hiking trails

Just about anywhere you go—north, south, east, or west—you're going to run into streams, trails, and outdoor activity areas. Also, this is a good area for gold panning.

Disc golf course

This is where we first got hooked on disc golf. We didn't realize, until we left, that this is considered a prime course—but we had always thought it was special.

Nevada County Fairgrounds

These fairgrounds are a cultural hub, from their Draft Horse Classic to their world music, bluegrass, and Celtic festivals, all set amongst tall pine trees and flower-lined walkways. There's something going on most weekends.

Lompoc, CA

My hometown tends to be on the quieter side, as it's off Hwy 101, along Scenic Hwy 1. Traveling from the south (Santa Barbara) toward Lompoc, you'll meander along Hwy 1 through areas that look much as they did a hundred years ago, sans the longhorn cattle. Cows still dot the brilliant green hillsides, which turn a soft golden velour in the summer and fall. Heading to Lompoc from the east (Buellton/Solvang), you'll feel as though you're winding through the hillsides of Italy. This is the world-renowned wine area known as the Santa Rita Appellation. Traveling from the north (San Luis Obispo), you may catch a glimpse of the brilliant light from a recently launched missile from Vandenburg Air Force Base, or hear the rumble and bang of its sonic boom.

Lompoc Points of Interest:

La Purisima Mission

This is one of the largest restoration projects accomplished by the Civilian Conservation Corps (CCC). Unlike many missions, La Purisima has not been encroached upon by civilization, thus the setting is much as it would've been in the early 1800s, including native, herbal, and vegetable gardens.

Whether you prefer walking through the native plant gardens, taking pictures of big horned sheep, or having a picnic next to the fountains, you'll leave more relaxed than you came. Check out their night tours, reenactment days, mountain men rendezvous, and even ghost tours. This area is a hot spot for paranormal investigators.

Old Town

This historic area is in the process of gentrifying. Here you'll find a charming coffee shop, a posh tea shop, loads of antiques and collectibles at great prices, and classy clothing. Wine tasting, tapas, and music liven up the night.

Murals

Lompoc is known as a mural town. We have loads of murals, painted by locals, nationally-known artists, and volunteers. I was honored to work on our first mural-in-a-day, back in the early 1990s; and from there they've been growing every year. Stop by the Chamber of Commerce to get a mural brochure, or check them out online.

Surf Beach

Ten miles west of town, you'll find Ocean Park and, just past that, Surf Beach. Here you can play in the soft sand, observe the wild surf, and even catch the Amtrak train. See the bird refuge and learn about local wildlife from Ocean Park. There are also some amazing sea caves, south of the train station, which can be reached during certain times of the year.

The Wine Ghetto and wineries

Yep, I said wine "ghetto" not "grotto." New wine tasting rooms are popping up all over this city of arts and flowers. The wine ghetto is an industrial park on the outskirts of town that has cleverly turned itself into a collection of tasting rooms. Don't let the industrial look fool you—inside each tasting room, you'll find a unique vibe.

Disc golf course

Recently a group of locals got together and put in a nice, eighteen-hole disc golf course with moveable pin positions. This course is situated at the picturesque Beattie park. Even if you don't play disc golf, this park is a great place to spend an afternoon and watch our brilliant sunsets.

Solvang

This Danish town, about thirty minutes east of Lompoc, was settled in 1911 by Danes escaping the intense Midwest winters. This is a tourist hot spot and a fun place to spend the day shopping, wine or brew tasting, bakery hopping, gelato tasting, or just relaxing in the park, watching passers-by. Visit a local institution, The Book Loft, for just about any kind of book and a cappuccino on your way to the Hans Christian Andersen museum.

Los Olivos and Los Alamos

Both of these charming towns are often used to film old movies. If you love horses, art, wine, flatbread pizza, or just cool little old towns, these are a must-visit. Los Olivos is a bit more refined, while smaller Los Alamos has an older, more rustic charm.

Santa Barbara, CA

In Santa Barbara, we had trouble finding our own short-term rental unit, so we camped for a bit then decided to just stay an hour away in Lompoc. While Peter was on this travel assignment, I worked as a personal assistant for an art instructor.

Santa Barbara is a unique city, nestled between the mountains and the ocean, with a pleasant warm Mediterranean weather pattern. It's expensive to stay there, but it's beautiful, with its Spanish colonial style and pretty beaches. Did I mention the beautiful scenery, art, music, theater, great trails for hiking, and biking, etc.?

Ritzy Santa Barbara is also full of very inquisitive patients. In the outpatient clinic, these knowledgeable folks wanted to know exactly which muscle was being worked and why. This is a great place to keep you on your toes, so keep a reference book on hand if you're a bit rusty.

Santa Barbara Points of Interest:

State Street

Lower and middle State Street are the tourist hubs. Even past locals like us like to stroll this vibrant area and stop into Dargan's Irish pub for a pint, after a tasty dinner at Flavor of India on upper State.

Stearns Wharf

Each time we come to Santa Barbara, we have to visit the wharf, at least to get a chocolate turtle at the candy shop. Sometimes we have fresh fish upstairs at the Longboard's Grill and watch the boats, pelicans, and seagulls dance across the soft swells. It's pretty magical at sunset.

Santa Barbara Harbor

Here you'll find yet more scrumptious seafood on which to dine. Walk off your dinner by wandering and checking out the boats in the harbor, view scuttling crabs along the harbor rocks, and stroll to the little strand at the end of the paved path.

Santa Barbara Botanical Gardens

This seventy-eight acre garden with five and a half miles of trails keeps you busy looking at all the new wonders that pop up each season. In the heat of the day, the sweet smells of sagebrush and wild flowers perfume the air, while the babbling stream and chirping birds erase any stress with their relaxing music.

Hiking, camping, beaches, and more

There are just too many outdoor activities to list, but suffice it to say that the tourist information, Internet, and Chamber of Commerce will give you guidance to exactly what you are looking for.

Santa Barbara Natural History Museum and Santa Barbara Museum of Art

Pleasantly wile away a day perusing the chock-full Natural History Museum. There's always something new for all ages, and its natural setting makes it a beautiful and aromatic place for a picnic.

Back in town, the Museum of Art is located right on State Street, so you can wander the halls, have lunch at their café, and continue your sight-seeing, all without driving anywhere.

Two fine disc golf courses

Just like Texas, California is now filling up with disc golf courses, and this area is no exception with two courses just outside of Santa Barbara, in Isla Vista and in Goleta.

OREGON

Eugene, OR

We were in awe of Eugene's huge library, resplendent with a coffee shop and used bookstore. Just near this library is the city bus depot, which made getting around easy. We also took full advantage of Eugene's plentiful bike paths, especially the Willamette River bike trail. On weekends, we explored the little towns all around, including those up the Colombia river. Check out the Eugene Folk Festival!

While Peter worked in different facilities in town and an hour away in Roseberg, I worked for Eugene's Juvenile Detention Center. It was an interesting experience, passing through multiple locked-down doors every day on my way to the office.

Toward the end of the traveling contract, the company set us up in hotels and a retirement manor along the Oregon coast for short assignments at their other facilities—a fun adventure.

Lincoln City, OR

We did a short stint here and stayed in a charming little apartment inside a retirement manor—a beautiful old building. The only drawback was having to watch our weight from their yummy all-inclusive dining room.

Newport, OR

Working a few days here just wasn't enough. We had to go back to take in the historical district in its entirety. I still remember the amazing crab cakes and Guinness ice cream at one of the restaurants along the harbor.

Roseburg, OR

This is an up-and-coming city with a large old town that seems to be awakening nicely from a long slumber.

Oregon Points of Interest

Oregon Coast

We traveled up the coast from Coos Bay to Astoria. Each one of the little coastal towns has its own unique flavor, so there was always something interesting to check out. Just before you get to the *hugantically* long bridge stretching across the Colombia River that connects Oregon with Washington's Olympic Penninsula (Astoria-Megler Bridge), you'll find yourself in the little town of Astoria. This charming community feels like a miniaturized version of San Francisco, with its steep streets and tall, narrow homes. It so charmed one of our traveler friends that she bought a home and settled there.

Hood River

We spent some time exploring this community as we toured alongside the Columbia River. On the way to Hood River, we stopped for lots of waterfall picnics and photo opportunities. If you're interested in year-round outdoor recreation, this is the place to visit.

Exploring the bigger cities

Although we drove through some of the larger cities, we didn't get enough time in any of them to get a feel for each place. We've heard wonderful things about Portland but never made it there.

WASHINGTON

After a job opportunity fell through in northern Washington, we followed a lead to Idaho. A few hours outside of Cour d'alene, Idaho, our recruiter called with bad news. It would take three months to get an Idaho license. Well, after our initial panic session, we just treated the drive as a reconnoiter mission, for future job possibilities. We had a nice visit in **Coeur d'Alene** and stayed the night in a mini-cabin at the Lake Coeur d'Alene Camping Resort. That night, they showed movies outside, and we discovered something new to us—a fresh popcorn-making vending machine!

The next day, we headed west back to Washington. We stopped along the way to get more camping gear. We wanted to be picky about our next assignment, so we prepared to hunker down and camp for the long haul. We investigated a job in historic Mount Vernon, but at the last minute, they hired a non-traveler. Since we'd been enjoying this area of Washington, we decided to follow another nearby lead on Washington's **Olympic Peninsula**. Here we camped for ten days, just outside an amazingly un-rainy town called **Sequim**.

In Sequim, we patronized the local coffee shop, toured the lavender farms, and read up on the town's history. All the while, we continued to investigate job possibilities in Port Angeles and surrounding areas. Not one to miss an adventure, we caught a ferry from **Port Angeles** to **Victoria, Canada**.

After our ten days of camping, we ended up heading back to California for an opening in Santa Barbara. Washington ended up being a nice vacation, and we ended that vacation by being invited to a scrumptious fresh salmon fry.

Washington Points of Interest

Sequim (Squim)

This little gem sits in the shadow of Mount Olympia in what is known as the Blue Hole. The Blue Hole also encompasses British Columbia, for it's in the shadow of the great mountain. These areas are protected from a majority of the gray drizzly days. In Seattle, just two hours east, you'll get about 37 inches of rain per year, and **Forks**— just two hours west of Sequim and known to fans of the *Twilight* series—you'll find a temperate rainforest with upwards of 140 inches! Yet Sequim only receives about 15 inches or less of rain per year, which explains its many fragrant lavender farms.

Port Townsend

A classy little port community and tourist destination spot. A friend of ours recently move to Port Townsend permanently, and she feels as if she's still on vacation.

Port Angeles

This more rustic, up-and-coming port community is where many come to catch the ferry to Victoria, British Columbia. Remember to bring your passport, even for this short ferry ride to Canada.

Cashmere

This little town sits on the east side of the Cascades and is home to the fruit jellied candy that you've probably seen sold all over the country. Even if you're not a fan of fruit and nut confections, this little town is worth a night's stay to wander through the pretty old town, bakery, antique stores, and old-timey soda shop.

Leavenworth

On the edge of extinction, a community deep in the Cascade mountains reinvented themselves as an Alpine Bavarian Village. This community has a charm and spirit that attracts folks from all over. I was very impressed by what a group of community-minded locals could accomplish.

NEW MEXICO

We found New Mexico to be an enchanting, friendly, and relaxed state, in general. This was one of our all-time favorite places. It wasn't just one area we were enthralled with—it was just about everywhere we went! And we still want to go back, because there's so much more to experience.

Santa Fe, NM

This is the one place we almost settled down in and made our permanent residence. Santa Fe is a world destination spot for the arts. The blend of Native American and Spanish cultures adds a richness of community as well as a strong family-oriented vibe. The majority of employees in any store we shopped treated us with friendliness and patience. We wondered if this was due to the more laid-back way of life, even more laid-back than California's Central Coast! (Note: When the light turns green, don't rush into the intersection because there might be a few cars still meandering through the red light.)

Don't miss a walk up Canyon Road during the Christmas season. Bundle up in warm clothes and slip-resistant shoes, then join the throng of visitors in the town square and up Canyon Road. Canyon Road will be lined with *luminarias* (paper bag lanterns) and *farolitos* (open fires). Hot drinks can be found in galleries, along the street, and in coffee shops. The magical feeling is further enhanced by the art gallieries' light displays and festive decorations.

Santa Fe Points of Interest

Abiquiu (Abi-Q)

I can't say enough about this area. For one thing, it encompasses our all-time favorite New Mexico spot, the Ghost Ranch, as well as so much more. The greater Abiquiu area is home to many artists and a fabulous studio tour each year. Just up the highway from Bode's store (the store that has it all) sits another treasure—a once-abandoned pueblo that was given by Spain to a group of people called Genízaro, a mix of Spanish and Native American tribes. This community is known as the Village of Abiquiu.

One day we set out from Santa Fe to find the village. In Abiquiu, just past and across the highway from Bode's store, we began winding our way up a hill, nodding to the post office on our right and watching for cars on the narrow road. After a short drive, the narrow road dumped us out into a large hard-packed dirt lot. On one side of this lot sat a quiet and beautiful adobe Catholic church.

Although at this point we didn't know the Village of Abiquiu was a private community, the quiet homes around the circumference of the lot made us feel as if we should just back out the way we'd come. But then we saw, gracing the front of one home, a hand-painted sign stating, "Private Tourist, Galleria, Map, OPEN."

Peter, being made of sterner stuff than me, walked up to the wooden screen door and knocked. After a short wait, a tall gentleman with twinkling blue eyes welcomed us in.

We were meeting the well-known Napoleón Garcia, Sr., a published author and a wonderful storyteller.

We learned all about the village and the one exception that was made to enable a non-family member to own a residence there. The late artist Georgia O'Keeffe was allowed to buy an 18th-century compound near the center of the village. If you spend time with Napoleón (we visited often), he might even make you a tortilla on his old oven, a hand-me-down from O'Keeffe. (Note: When registering for a tour of her home through the Georgia O'Keeffe Museum in Santa Fe, plan early—it can take three or more months to get reservations.)

Ghost Ranch

We spent many weekends in this sublime area, mostly during the cooler off-seasons. We'd camp along the arroyo and take advantage of the camping area's indoor food prep and bathhouse. Then we'd wander down a little trail to the ranch's retreat area and have a self-serve lunch for a nominal fee. After a tour of the old buildings where Georgia O'Keeffe had visited and stayed, we'd head for the hills for a nice hike, grab a cup of tea or coffee, and peruse the Georgia O'Keeffe library or browse the gift store for cool tidbits to send home.

The colors in New Mexico astounded us but most especially around the Ghost Ranch. The mountains, horizontally striped in pastel sorbet hues, and the brilliant, bold ultramarine and cobalt skies were like walking into a Georgia O'Keeffe painting. Even in the midst of winter's snow, the Ghost Ranch was a captivating place to camp and explore. Note the little cabin near the entrance, which was built for the film *City Slickers*.

Taos

This is another artist delight of sights, sounds, and beauty. Charming shops and art galleries abound. Visit the largest standing multistory Pueblo structure in North America, the Taos Pueblo. Be respectful when visiting, as Pueblo Native Americans still live there.

Bradbury Science Museum in Los Alamos

Here you'll read all about nuclear energy, both how it assists us in today's world as well as the terror that it has unleashed. The information is surprising in its honesty. After a morning at the museum, you can grab some lunch at the local deli and enjoy the large park in the middle of town.

Las Vegas & Pecos National Historic Park

Las Vegas is a small town with a historic old town and square. Just outside of this community is the Pecos National Historic Park. The park's a nice place for easy walks to ruins of a Native American pueblo, including renovated underground rooms (kivas). Near Christmas, powdery white snow lines walkways that glitter and glow with hundreds of luminarias.

Bandelier National Monument

These surprisingly accessible cliff dwellings—after a bit of a drive—are full of history from those who lived and celebrated in these cliffs and the community below. Dogs are not allowed on these guided tours, but there are water and nicely shaded, chain link kennels available for them to relax in while you're touring.

Roswell

On our way from Texas to Santa Fe, we stopped in Roswell. Our stopover happened to coincided with the annual UFO Convention. The town was in full swing: Wal-mart's greeter was a giant green alien; along the sidewalk, the Coca-Cola machine sported a green alien knocking back a Coke; and even a local church played along, with a message that read, "Is Jesus alien to you?"

We wandered into the UFO museum, listened to some interesting talks, bought some Area 51 parking stickers, and headed to the ***Carlsbad Caverns.*** The caves were amazing, and I kept feeling as if I had to speak quietly, as though I were walking through a great cathedral. The air that far underground was surprisingly cool even when it was sweltering top-side.

Chama

Near the border of New Mexico and Colorado sits the tiny town of Chama. Here we caught the ***Cumbres and Toltec Scenic Railroad*** and traveled through the splendorous Rockies, stopping at the top for a delicious hot lunch. This is an amazing nature experience you'll not want to miss!

Pagosa Springs and Mesa Verde National Park, CO

While working in Santa Fe, we took a long weekend and explored parts northeast, into Colorado. ***Pagosa Springs*** is a pleasant little town—with hot springs bubbling up between the rocks along the river, right in the middle of town! From here we spent the day cruising to Mesa Verde, with a stop-over in Durango. We arrived at ***Mesa Verde National Park*** just in time to catch the last tour. We stayed the night at the top of the mesa, at the Far View Lodge, so we could start back to the ruins at first light. The lodge was nice, basic, and clean, with beautiful views. As a bonus for staying at the park, we got to see the sunrise and didn't have to navigate the steep drive up and down more than once! (I'm not fond of heights.) Make sure to take lots of water on your hikes, especially in the summer. (We do most of our exploring in the off-seasons, when it tends to be quieter and cooler.)

Sky City

On our way back to New Mexico from California, we stopped at this pueblo, which sits atop a high mesa. Only a few locals live here year-round due to the extremes in temperatures, although many still have homes up here. Even in the cold season, there were a few artisans in front of the adobe homes selling their pottery. The beautiful black and orange-painted pottery made by these Acoma Native Americans are revered throughout the country. The tour leaves from the visitors' center and cruises up the steep hillside—you have a choice to ride back down or hike down the old trails. As you wander this 'city in the sky' with your guide, you'll get a feel for what life might have been like in bygone days. You'll hear about their spiritual and communal ways, as well as the history of their pueblo and where they moved from. Some of the guides' stories will make you chuckle, while others will move you.

The views are amazing, and below the mesa, there's a nice coffee shop, an area where you can buy art from the local artisans, and also a gift shop.

Silver City, NM

Once this area was home to the Puebloan cultures, then to the Apache, the Spaniards, and later the American prospectors. Now this is a culturally diverse town of about 10,000 people. Here you'll also find the **Western New Mexico University**, founded in the late 1800s. The old town community is colorful and fun. In this historical district, you'll find little gems, from Yada Yada Yarn's dynamic knitters to The Curious Kumquat's amazing meals, and the yummy gelato at Alotta Gelato. Along with coffee shops and art galleries, you'll find some hip little stores. Copper mining is still the main industry here, and if you like historic communities, you'll enjoy this area.

Check out the deep crevice running through the center of the downtown area and the clever way the community put it to good use as a park. Keep your eyes peeled for top-quality musical groups who use this area as a stop over while on tour. And keep your ears open for the many proficient local Celtic musicians.

This area sits in one of the country's largest national wildernesses, **Gila National Forest**. Amazing Native American ruins, hot springs, and beautiful scenery can be found here. We spent every available moment exploring, walking, hiking, camping, and eating. Here we saw critters totally new to us: Coatimundi, *javelina* (also known as "jabalina" or "peccary"), beautiful blue cicada, and a vinegaroon.

One of the friendly folks at the local nursing home, where Peter worked, invited us to spend Christmas with their big extended family. We laughed and chatted over homemade pasole, brews, and treats. This was a special gift we will never forget.

Silver City Points of Interest:

Shakespeare Ghost Town

This privately-owned mining town of old is refreshing in its non-commercialized simplicity. This place really takes you back without romanticizing the message. It looks as though Billy the Kid made it here, as well. He seems to have lived everywhere in these parts, including Silver City.

Pinos Altos

Walking around this community, just outside of Silver City, you'll feel as though you're back in the mid to late 1800s. Enjoy a quality meal at the Buckhorn Saloon and Opera House, a destination spot for people as far north as Albuquerque. Take in a melodrama next door and learn the history of Gila National Forest's locals like Geronimo from the chock-full museum. Visit the Hearst Methodist Church built in 1898 by the Hearst family of newspaper fame. It's now home to the Grant County Art Guild.

Mogollon (mug-ee-own)

On a weekend drive, north of Silver City, we stopped in the tiny, former mining town of Mogollon. We visited during the monsoon season, and all was lush and green. An unexpected delight was finding a little coffee shop. Here we grabbed hot drinks then wandered the town and chatted up the locals.

Gila National Forest

This was Apache territory—a beautiful wilderness area peppered with streams, hot springs, trails, hidden surprises, and quiet Native American ruins. The Native American cliff dwellings are well preserved and the scenic drive and walk to access them is an added bonus. This area is also where the Mexican gray wolf has been reintroduced into the environment, amongst both smiles and trepidation.

One night in Silver City, during a huge moon that sat low and full, Peter saw four gray wolves glide across the road, backlit by the moon. What a sight to behold!

The City of Rocks State Park

Groups of enchanting, tall stones congregate as if carefully placed by unknown hands, giving the park its other name, Natural Stonehenge. This was another of our favorite places to camp. We'd lie against the warm rocks, after sunset, watching for shooting stars against the velvet black sky. See if you can spot a coatimundi or a brilliant blue cicada when you visit.

Catwalk

Don't miss this Civilian Conservation Core (CCC) restoration project. You'll walk along metal-grated walkways, hoof it up grated stairs and across a swinging bridge over musical waterfalls and serene streams. Wave to goats on the hill-side as you weave through the rocky cliffs.

White Sands, NM

This is the first time I'd ever experienced warm snow! Well, it was sand, but the white was so brilliant, it looked like snow. As this was our pup's first experience with sand, she was a bit confused that this white substance didn't cause her feet to freeze. But soon she took to it like a fish to water.

Tombstone, Arizona

We took a long weekend while in Silver City to explore this region. *(See more under Arizona)*.

Palomas, Chihuahua (Mexico)

Another weekend trip, this time just south of Silver City, found us in this tiny, Mexican town. Check out the friendly folks at The Pink Store and Restaurant, and ponder the Poncho Villa and Lt./Gen. Patton connection.

TEXAS

Fredericksburg, TX

An hour north of San Antonio, in the Texas hill country, sits a community founded by German Freethinkers. The old architectural styles were completely new to us and had us intrigued. The very thick walls of some of the older buildings kept them nice and cool even in the heat of summer. Here we were introduced to our first catfish fry, spiced bugs (crawfish/crawdad), summer hail, and the most incredible lightening storms.

I found a job working on a new computer system for the local health food store, The Peach Basket. This store became our go-to place for our grocery shopping, and the little coffee shop next door was another favorite. We enjoyed our short four-month contract here exploring, wine tasting, and indulging in all the great food. It was also a great jumping-off point for visiting Austin and San Antonio.

Texas Points of Interest:

The Alamo

I never understood why Texas seemed like its own country until now. We learned the multicultural history of Texas and about the folks, from all over the world, who fought together to make it theirs. It's best to visit the Alamo with a dyed-in-the-wool Texan to get a more animated story of the Alamo's history, since they've been taught about it since childhood. We also happened to visit during a reenactment day, so everyone was in the uniform and regalia of the Alamo's heyday.

River Walk

Whenever we mention we were in San Antonio, everyone wants to know if we made it to the River Walk. Yep, and it is a very clever and beautiful use of their waterways. While walking along the River Walk in the thick, heavy heat, we looked longingly at those gracefully floating down the little river. Next time, we vowed, we'd be viewing the river walk from that perspective.

Bandera

This little bayou town is touted as the 'Cowboy Capital of the World.' After lunch and dessert under the watchful eyes of the stuffed jackalope, we walked it off with a stroll down to the park lining the Medina River. Bring your camera, especially in the springtime, because everywhere you go, you'll find a *Kodak moment*.

New Braunfels

Since the hill country area was settled by German Free-thinkers, you'll see a lot of their influence, especially in the smaller towns. This place is famous for its huge water park (Schlitterbahn) and their amazing wursts (sausages).

Stonehenge II and Easter Island Heads

These are located a bit off the beaten path. Traveling there is a fun excursion, and it's a nice place to have a picnic lunch. You can enjoy the hill country, especially when the wild flowers are blooming, and see the creative use of artistic talent.

▸ Fun Places Traveled between Assignments

ALASKA

We caught a flight to **Anchorage,** our cruise jumping-off place, and spent the afternoon wandering the city. The little time we spent in Anchorage made us wish for a land vacation in their state parks. And yes, we did have to pull our shades against the perpetual twilight to get some sleep.

Our taxi driver told us that when the salmon were running, as they were at that time, the drivers would fish in the river that ran through town all through night then go back to driving all day. We were a bit leery about the quality of taxi service we'd get from exhausted drivers, but all went well. We only wished we had somewhere to cook the salmon they were selling.

From Anchorage, we caught our Carnival ship and headed down Alaska's Inside Passage. We were very happy we upgraded to a balcony room, as we spent a lot of time just watching the beautiful scenery and searching for bears.

On the land tours during the cruise, we learned all about the Russian influences in this part of the country. This helped us to better understand our own West-Coast history and why Spain had erected so many missions to protect the area from Russia. Our favorite place along the cruise route was **Juneau**. Not only is this the capital of Alaska, but it's also one of the few communities along the Inside Passage that hasn't burnt down. So the buildings still have their original historic charm. Just outside of town, we saw black bears and bald eagles. If we'd gone there in June when the salmon were running, we'd have seen orcas right from the middle of town!

Mendenhall glacier is a site I can't do justice with words. It seemed to glow as if it was backlit with a surreal cool blue light. It was a beautiful color that I'd never seen in nature.

CANADA

Our Alaskan cruise ended in **Vancouver**. There we took in a land tour and hit the highlights for our short time in the city. The 1000-plus acre **Stanley Park**, full of totem poles and beautiful grounds, was a sight to see. And of course we ate our way through **Granville Island**—loved their giant indoor food market!

CARIBBEAN

During the Christmas season in New Mexico, we took our first cruise. We met our San Antonio, TX, family and all carpooled down to **Galveston** and from there set out to sea. I was in awe of the differences in cultures in this part of the country, so I spent a lot of time just people-watching. Of course, I ate my way through the cruise, as well. We enjoyed our afternoon teas with petit fours and beautiful piano music. Then we wandered around, sampling the different music, wine, art, food, yoga, gym, sauna, and fun events. Most nights, there were very high-quality performances on the main stage.

We enjoyed our rum cake tasting in **Jamaica**, a sea turtle preserve in the **Cayman Islands**, and the cheerfully painted community of **Cozumel**. Our best time was in Cozumel, where we rented a car and traveled inland. Then we took a tour through the crocodile and turtle sanctuary. The folks in Cozumel were about the friendliest we'd met so far, and the sand was warm and beckoning. I did get wild and get a tattoo on my upper arm while relaxing on the beach. (Well, it was done in India ink, but I still felt reckless.) Also, you can rent snorkeling gear on the beach, but note that you'll be admonished if you touch the turtles swimming near.

On the last day, of our cruise Peter decided to play bingo and to buy some raffle tickets. He lost at bingo but won us an Alaskan cruise from the raffle tickets! Peter, Mr. Lucky, had also made some money at the casino the night before, so we were sitting pretty for our next adventure.

ENGLAND

London, Peter's native home, is an old land, filled with rich history, lush green foliage, and lots to do. In bustling London, we took the Underground everywhere. We did a whirlwind tour between visits to old cemeteries, Roman ruins, Celtic ruins, old forests, **Stonehenge**, **The Cotswold**, **Isle of Wight**, and **Bath.** On our last few days, we caught a bus to the castled city of **Cardiff, Wales**. Here, at a Celtic reenactment village, we learned about the forefathers of the modern Welsh—the Celts. England is also where I found my love of dark, rich, locally-brewed beer, which could be had in any pub, along side fish and chips and jacket potatoes.

GERMANY

Upon landing, we lamented the drastic change of scenery as we set our eyes in the sterile, industrial Frankfurt airport after two weeks in green and charmingly historic England. But, just after leaving the industrial airport, the local charm of the area began to unveil itself as we cruised to **Ludwigshafen am Rhein**, my father-in-law's hometown. Here we enjoyed family reunions. Here also I learned what it was to be a foreigner—something everyone should experience at least once—since many of the older folks didn't speak English, and our German was almost nonexistent.

In Germany, we ate Greek food and quantities of gelato with fresh fruit served by tuxedo-clad Italians. We took a quick trip over to **Strasbourg, France**, where we were serenaded by our waiter as he brought our flammenkuchen (pizza-like meal) whilst singing "Born to be Wild" and tossing a treat to the pup following close on his heals. After lunch, we visited the awe-inspiring **Strasbourg cathedral**, followed by a relaxing water cruise around the city.

Back in Germany, we spent a day being charmed by **Heidelberg Castle** and the rich, colorful tulips all around Ludwigshafen.

After returning to the States, I tried to figure out what one blurry picture could be. Later, we realized Peter had taken a photo of his cousin's speedometer on the **Autoban**. It was equal to a *modest* 125 mph. Even at that speed, other drivers had been easily sailing past us.

IRELAND

It's true what they say about there being forty shades of green in Ireland. Just off the plane, we immediately wandered around medieval ***Dublin***, where we filled our camera with shot after shot before looking for a place to turn in. Word to the wise—staying in a hostel in the center of Dublin after a long flight isn't the best idea. There's a reason the Irish call this area 'England West.' Locals say it's where the French and English come to party. All around our room, there was lots of partying into the wee hours of the morn. Once with blurry, jet-lagged eyes, we peered out our door to see folks lying about in the hallway, singing colorful French songs and knocking back more than a wee dram of spirits.

We could've spent a week just walking and experiencing Dublin and its rich history. At the 47-acre **Trinity College**, we met friendly folks who called around to help us locate one of my pet projects—finding the Irish connection to my Choctaw tribe. I'd heard that there was a plaque commemorating our chief's visit to Ireland but had been unable to locate any more information.

The Trinity staff weren't sure where this plaque was but believed it was further west, so we hopped a bus and headed that way. We stopped in and explored **Galway** and **Castlebar**. Then in **Westport**, the end of the line for the bus, we were directed as far west as we could go, to the coastal village of **Louisburgh**. A quiet, elderly taxi driver drove us the distance while his radio played soothing old-time American rock and roll, something we'd come to expect in Ireland. That night, we stayed in one of the few B & Bs in the tiny town of Louisburgh.

When we got to town, we found only a few stores open. We wandered into the pharmacy and asked the owner if he knew about the Choctaw plaque. Hooray, the owner knew exactly what we were talking about! But sadly, the museum with this information was closed for the next few days. We were crushed but cheered back up when he told us that he'd call his friend Mary, whose cousin Mary managed the museum—Mary is a very popular name in Ireland.

Mary very kindly came down, opened the museum, and even made us tea and biscuits whilst settling us in front of a film about the namesake of this **Granuaile Visitor Centre**. This center, although mostly focused on the female pirate Granuaile, was also a museum for the Great Famine in Ireland. It was here I found the connection between my Choctaw relatives and the Irish. An entire display was devoted to the Choctaw people and their help during the Great Famine. They even had a pretty plaque dedicated to our then chief.

The next day, we caught a taxi back to Westport, where we hopped on a bus to the southernmost part of Ireland. The friendliness and hospitality of folks in the southern area was unrivaled. Even the bus drivers seem to be in a jovial mood. We took in the sights and wandered the **Ring of Kerry**, where friendly locals let us know why we should NOT kiss the **Blarney stone.** Local boys enjoy using it for target practice when their bladders are full.

We also met some interesting folks in a hostel in **Kilkenny** and at a B & B in **Kilarney**. One fun chap from New Zealand ended up as our travel companion until we parted ways in County Cork. Back in Dublin, we caught a bus north to **Dragheda** to the 5,000-year-old ancient temple, **Newgrange**. This was something mind expanding and so different from anything else we'd experienced.

The only regret we had for this visit is that we didn't get a chance to make it the Giant's Causeway in northern Ireland.

Things to note: You can easily get around with a backpack and public transportation. You'll need less clothes than you think, since you can hand wash and let them dry on the radiant heaters.

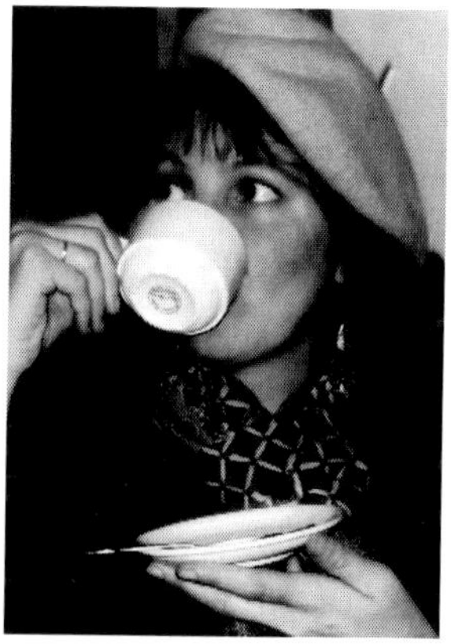

About the Author

Michelle Schaefer, is owner of Bohemian Spirit Design: a writing, publishing, fine art, and graphic design business. She, her husband, and their critters call Santa Barbara County their home base.

Schaefer's artistic and detective-like brain drives her love of research and study into the nature of... everything. And to that end she continues to type and illustrate her knowledge into easily accessible material for both lay folk and not-so-lay folk.

Upcoming books from the author: *Going Green on a Dime in Your Home*; *Going Green on a Dime in Your Garden*; *Ayurveda illustrated*; and *Feng Shui and Ayurvedic Interior Design*.

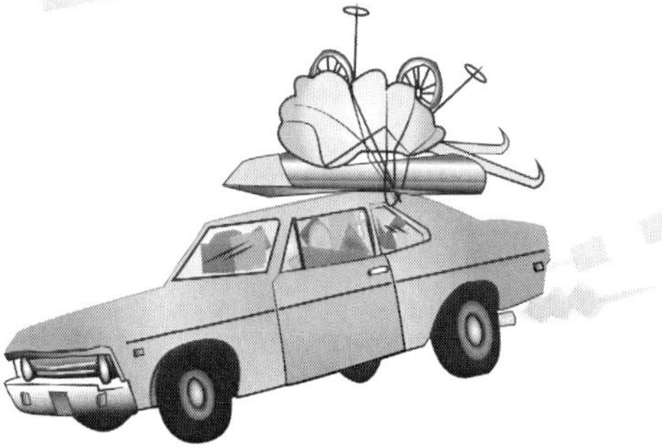

Made in United States
North Haven, CT
10 November 2026

22096552R00080

Get the full breakfast and then save the rest for lunch while you are on the road or out and about. Also remember: at restaurants, unlike in the U.S., you won't get your bill unless you ask for it. This is a sign of respect, as it shows they're not trying to rush you. Of course, we learned that lesson after a lot of waiting.

Through all our travels in Ireland, the audio memory that still plays in my brain is one that we heard on every public transportation bus we took: "Stand back... Luggage doors are op-por-rrrrating... Stand back... Luggage doors are ap-por-rrrrating!"